The Ultimate Dash Diet Dinner Recipes Cookbook

Burn Fats with a Collection of Easy and Affordable Recipes for Beginners

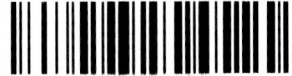

Maya Wilson

Table of contents

The Vegan Lovers Refried Beans

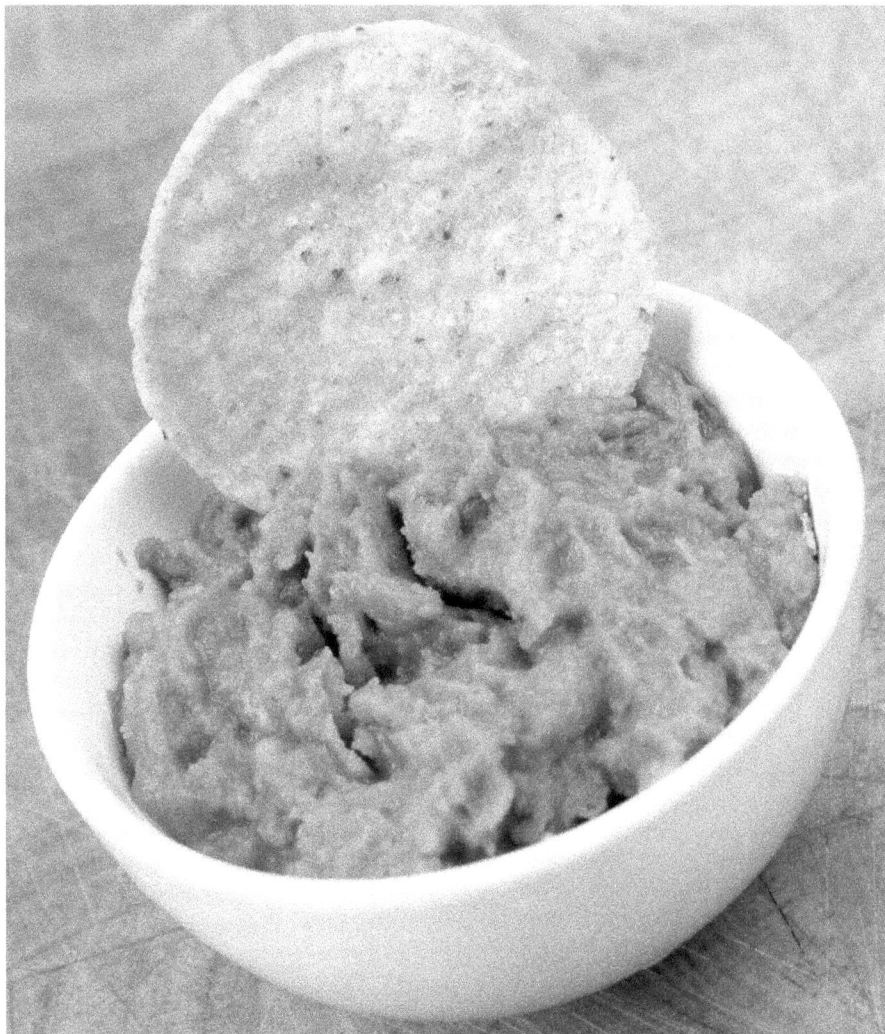

Serving: 12

Prep Time: 5 minutes

Cook Time: 10 hours

Ingredients:

- 4 cups vegetable broth

- 4 cups water

- 3 cups dried pinto beans

- 1 onion, chopped

- 2 jalapeno peppers, minced

- 4 garlic cloves, minced

- 1 tablespoon chili powder

- 2 teaspoon ground cumin

- 1 teaspoon sweet paprika
- 1 teaspoon salt
- ½ teaspoon fresh ground black pepper

How To:

1.   Add the listed ingredients to your Slow Cooker.

2.   Cover and cook on HIGH for 10 hours .

3.   If there's any extra liquid, ladle the liquid up and reserve it during a bowl .

4.   Use an immersion blender to blend the mixture (in the Slow Cooker) until smooth.

5.   Add the reserved liquid.

6.   Serve hot and enjoy!

Nutrition (Per Serving)

Calories: 91

Fat: 0g

Carbohydrates: 16g

Protein: 5g

Cool Apple and Carrot Harmony

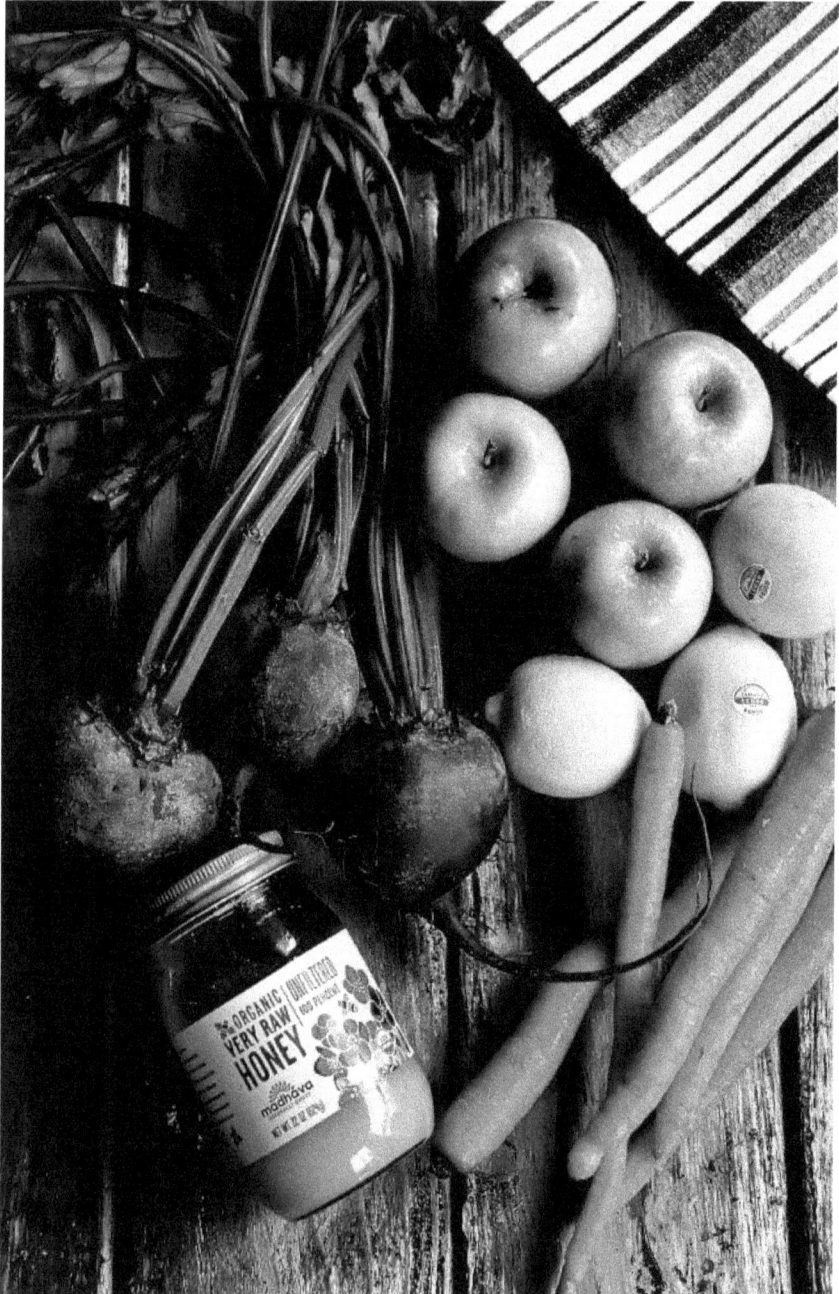

Serving: 6

Prep Time: 10 minutes

Cook Time: 10 minutes

Ingredients:

- 1 cup apple juice

- 1 pound baby carrots

- 1 tablespoon cornstarch

- 1 tablespoon mint, chopped

How To:

1. Add fruit juice , carrots, cornstarch and mint to your Instant Pot.

2. Stir and lock the lid.

3. Cook on high for 10 minutes.

4. Perform a fast release.

5. Divide the combination amongst plates and serve.

6. Enjoy!

Nutrition (Per Serving)

Calories: 161

Fat: 2g

Carbohydrates: 9g

Protein: 8g

Mac and Chokes

Serving: 6

Prep Time: 5 minutes

Cook Time: 20 minutes

Ingredients:

- 1 tablespoon of olive oil

- 1 large sized diced onion

- 10 minced garlic cloves

- 1 can artichoke hearts

- 1-pound uncooked macaroni shells

- 12-ounce baby spinach

- 4 cups vegetable broth

- 1 teaspoon red pepper flakes

- 4 ounces vegan cheese

- ¼ cup cashew cream

How To:

1.   Set the pot to Sauté mode and add oil, allow the oil to heat up and add onions.

2.   Cook for two minutes.

3.   Add garlic and stir well.

4.   Add artichoke hearts and sauté for 1 minute more.

5.   Add uncooked pasta and three cups of broth alongside 2 cups of water.

6.   Mix well.

7.   Lock the lid and cook on high for 4 minutes.

8.   Quick release the pressure.

9.   Open the pot and stir.

10.   Add extra water, fold in spinach and cook on Sauté mode for a couple of minutes.

11.   Add cashew cream and grated vegan cheese.

12.   Add pepper flakes and blend well.

13.   Enjoy!

Nutrition (Per Serving)

Calories: 649

Fat: 29g

Carbohydrates: 64g

Protein: 34g

Black Eyed Peas and Spinach Platter

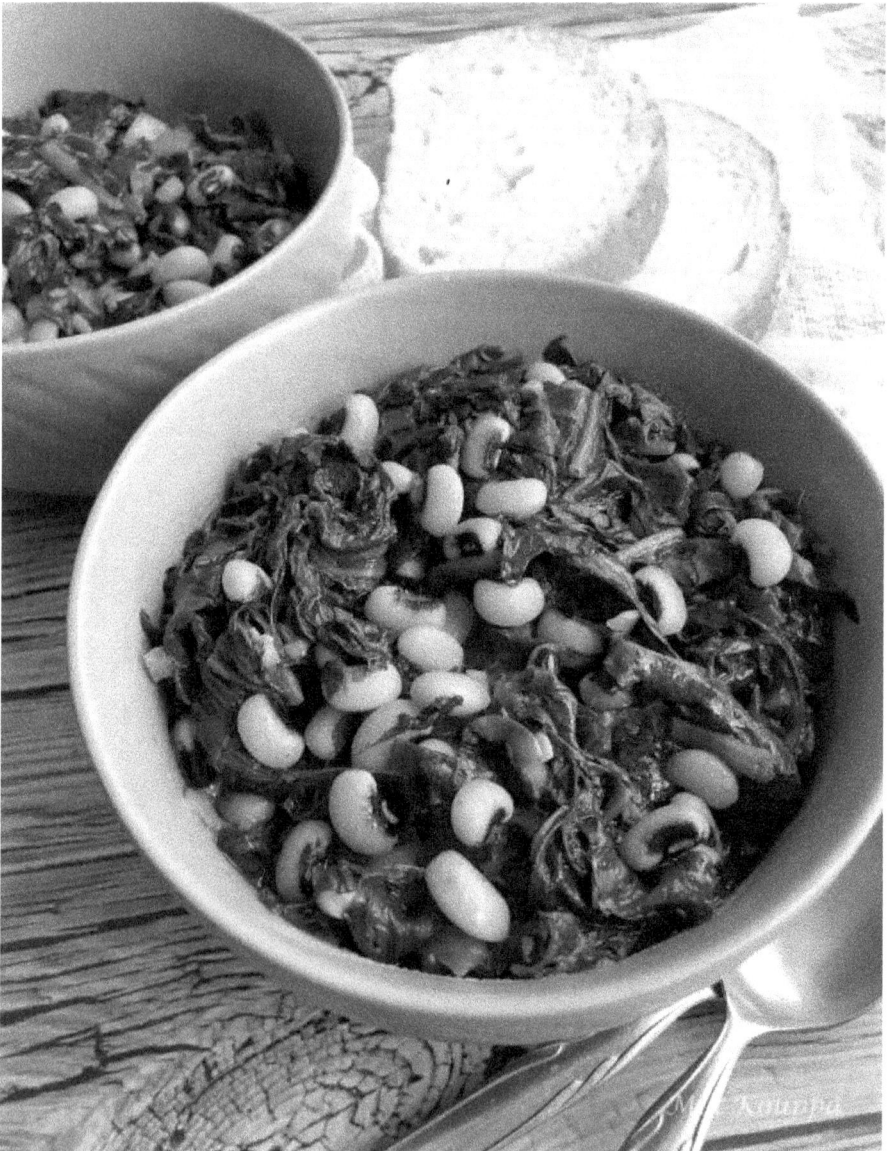

Serving: 4

Prep Time: 10 minutes

Cook Time: 8 hours

Ingredients:

- 1 cup black eyed peas, soaked overnight and drained

- 2 cups low-sodium vegetable broth

- 1 can (15 ounces) tomatoes, diced with juice

- 8 ounces ham, chopped

- 1 onion, chopped

- 2 garlic cloves, minced

- 1 teaspoon dried oregano

- 1 teaspoon salt

- ½ teaspoon freshly ground black pepper ½ teaspoon ground mustard 1 bay leaf

How To:

1.   Add the listed ingredients to your Slow Cooker and stir.

2.   Place lid and cook on LOW for 8 hours.
3.   Discard the herb .
4.   Serve and enjoy!

Nutrition (Per Serving)

Calories: 209

Fat: 6g

Carbohydrates: 22g

Protein: 17g

Humble Mushroom Rice

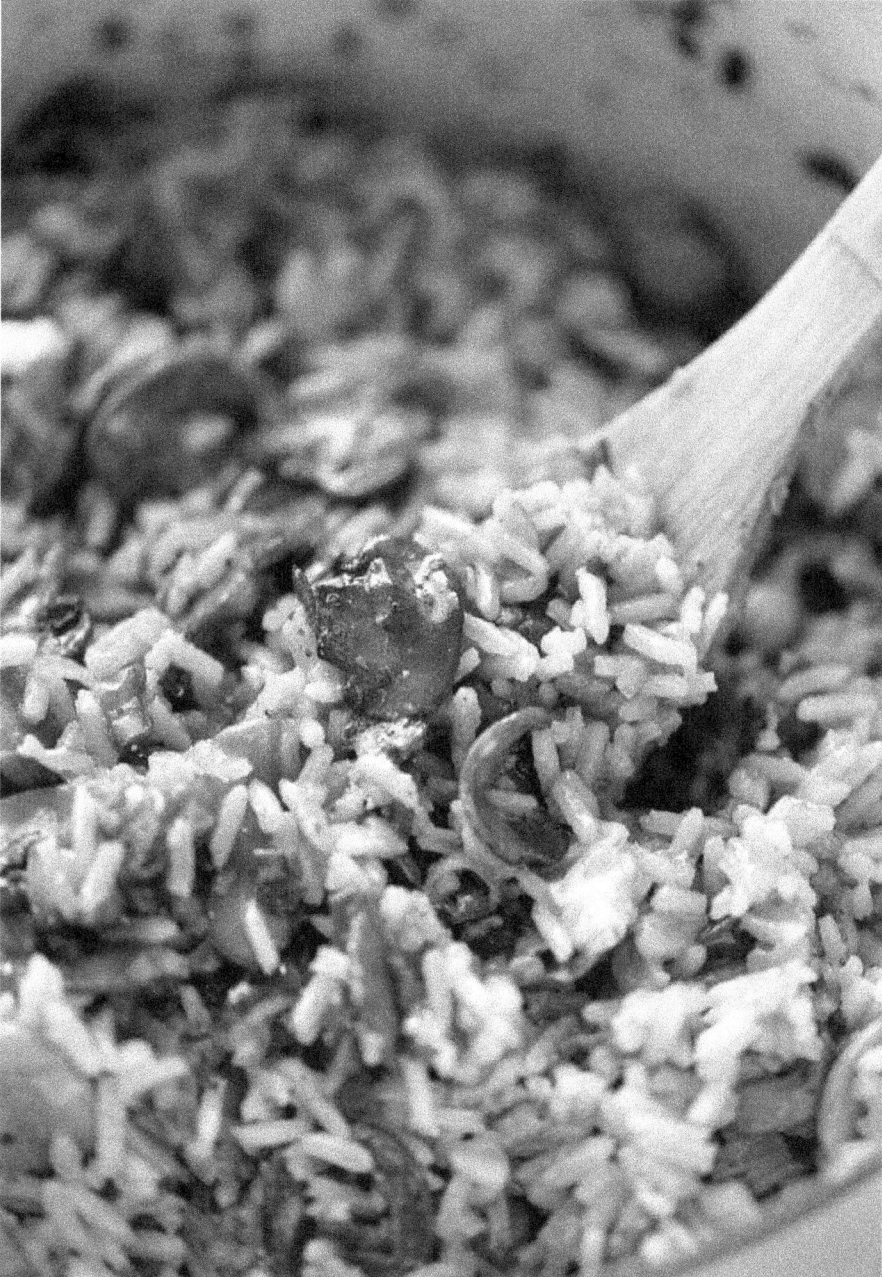

Serving: 3

Prep Time: 10 minutes

Cook Time: 3 hours

Ingredients:

- ½ cup rice

- 2 green onions chopped

- 1 garlic clove, minced

- ¼ pound baby Portobello mushrooms, sliced 1 cup vegetable stock

How To:

1. Add rice, onions, garlic, mushrooms, stock to your Slow Cooker.
2. Stir well and place lid.

3.   Cook on LOW for 3 hours..

4.   Stir and divide amongst serving platters.

5. Enjoy!

Nutrition (Per Serving)

Calories: 200

Fat: 6g

Carbohydrates: 28g

Protein: 5g

Sweet and Sour Cabbage and Apples

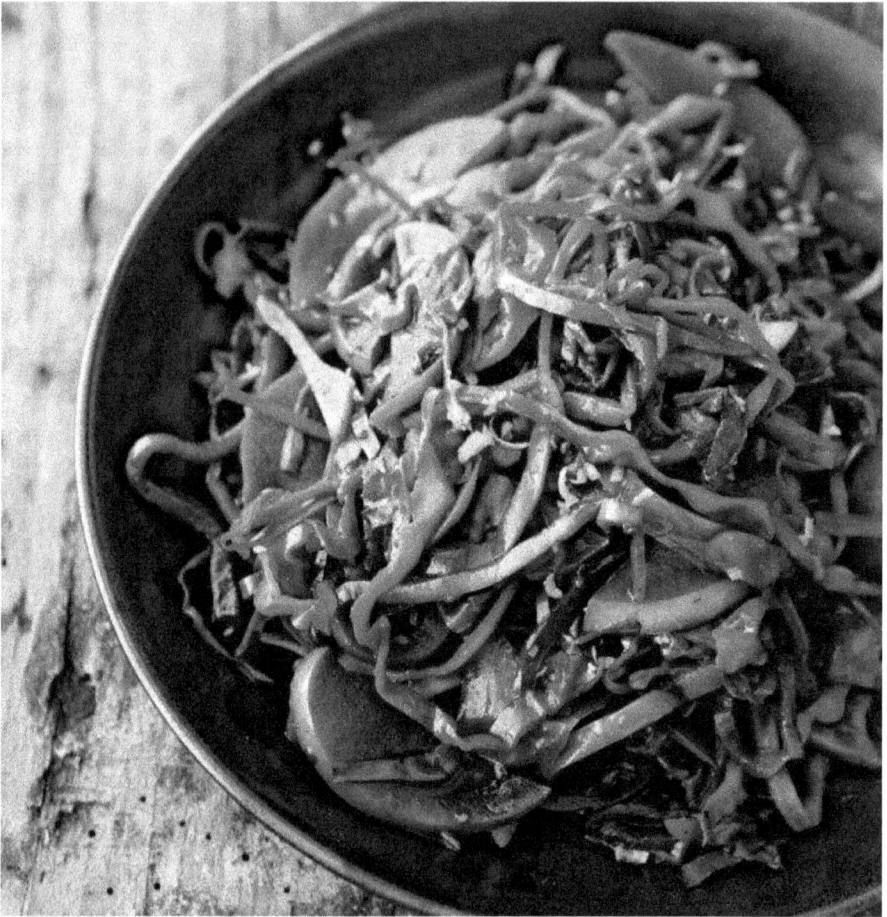

Serving: 4

Prep Time: 15 minutes

Cook Time: 8 hours

Ingredients:

- ¼ cup honey

- ¼ cup apple cider vinegar

- 2 tablespoons Orange Chili-Garlic Sauce

- 1 teaspoon sea salt

- 3 sweet tart apples, peeled, cored and sliced

- 2 heads green cabbage, cored and shredded

- 1 sweet red onion, thinly sliced

How To:

1.	Take alittle bowl and whisk in honey, orange-chili aioli , vinegar.

2.	Stir well.

3.	Add honey mix, apples, onion and cabbage to your Slow Cooker and stir.

4.	Close lid and cook on LOW for 8 hours.

5.	Serve and enjoy!

Nutrition (Per Serving)

Calories: 164

Fat: 1g

Carbohydrates: 41g

Protein: 4g

Delicious Aloo Palak

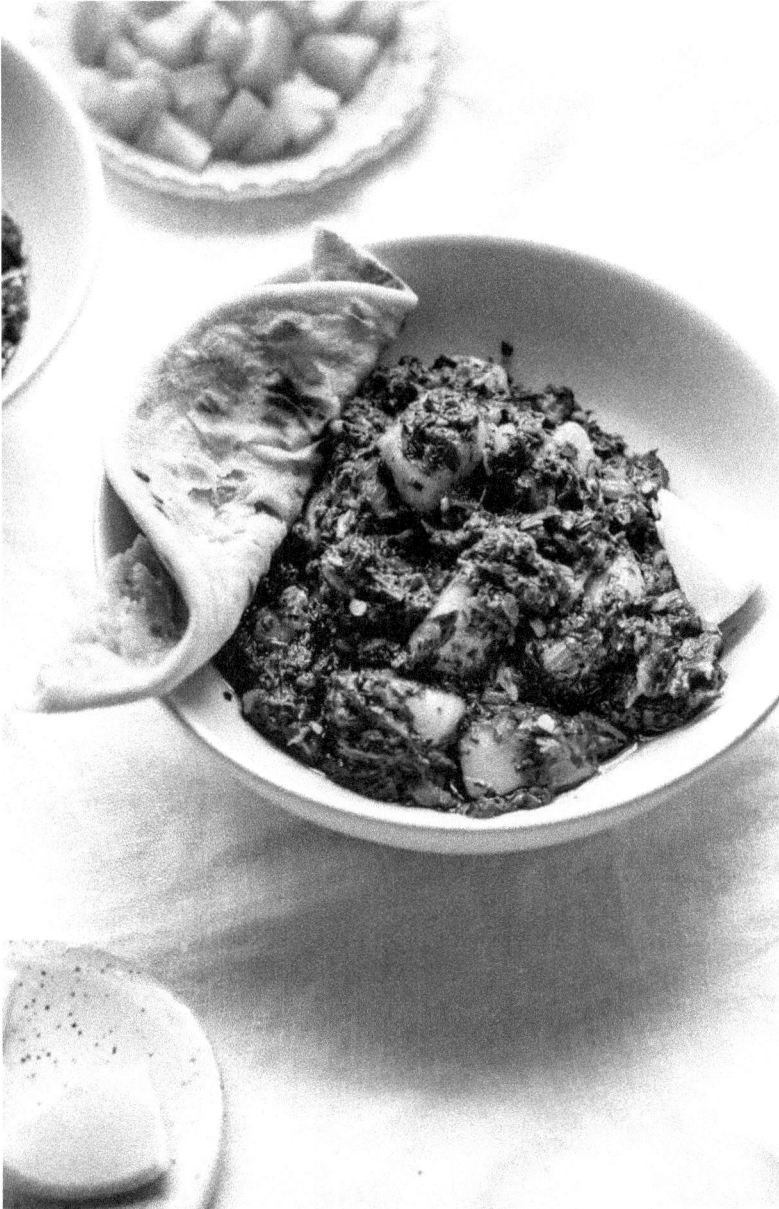

Serving: 6

Prep Time: 10 minutes

Cook Time: 6-8 hours

Ingredients:

- 2 pounds red potatoes, chopped

- 1 small onion, diced

- 1 red bell pepper, seeded and diced

- ¼ cup fresh cilantro, chopped

- 1/3 cup low-sodium veggie broth

- 1 teaspoon salt

- ½ teaspoon Garam masala
- ½ teaspoon ground cumin

- ¼ teaspoon ground turmeric

- ¼ teaspoon ground coriander

- ¼ teaspoon freshly ground black pepper 2 pounds fresh spinach, chopped

How To:

1.   Add potatoes, bell pepper, onion, cilantro, broth and seasoning to your Slow Cooker.

2.   Mix well.

3.   Add spinach on top.

4.   Place lid and cook on LOW for 6-8 hours.

5.   Stir and serve.

6.   Enjoy!

Nutrition (Per Serving)

Calories: 205

Fat: 1g

Carbohydrates: 44g

Protein: 9g

Orange and Chili Garlic Sauce

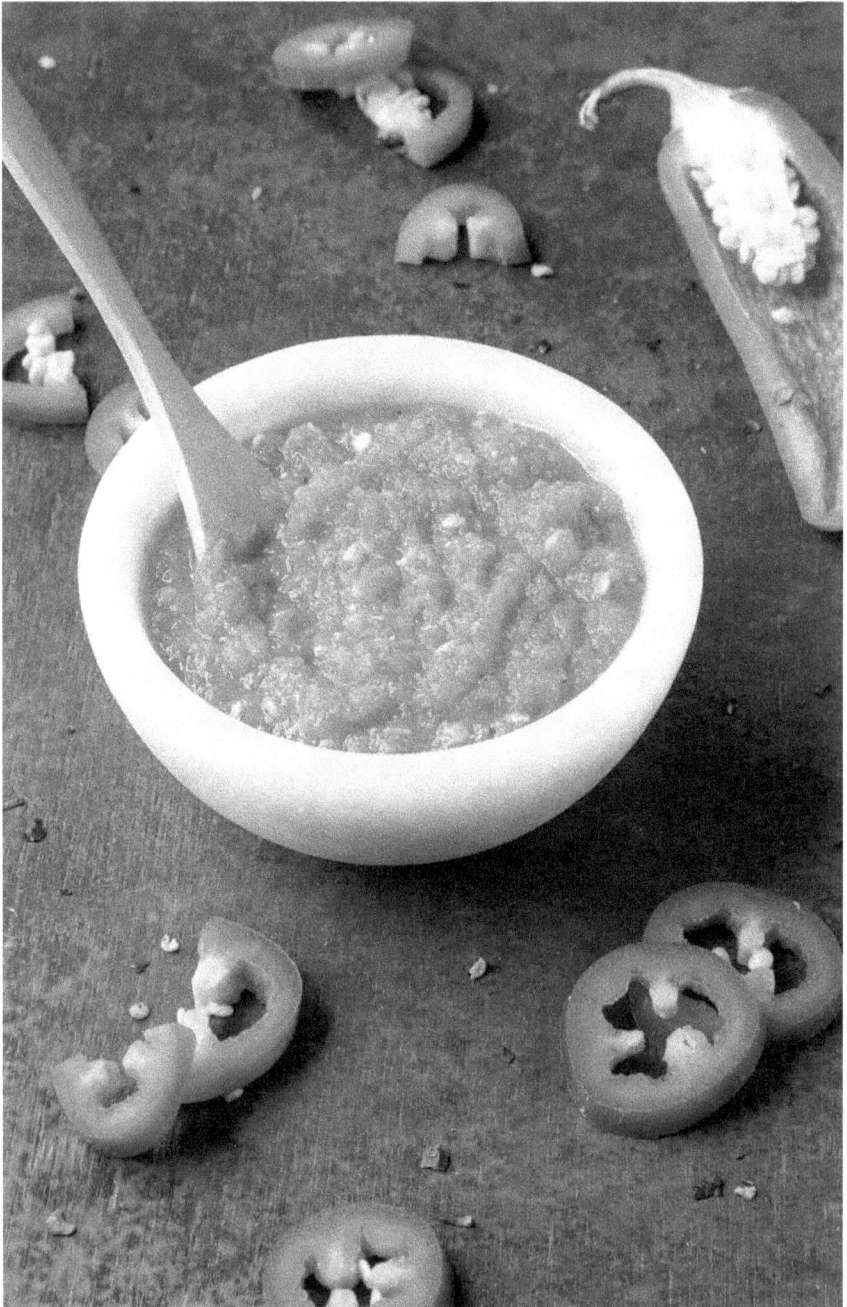

Serving: 5 cups

Prep Time: 15 minutes

Cook Time: 8 hours

Ingredients:

- ½ cup apple cider vinegar

- 4 pounds red jalapeno peppers, stems, seeds and ribs removed, chopped

- 10 garlic cloves, chopped

- ½ cup tomato paste

- Juice of 1 orange zest

- ½ cup honey

- 2 tablespoons soy sauce

- 2 teaspoons salt

How To:

1.   Add vinegar, garlic, peppers, ingredient , fruit juice , honey, zest, soy and salt to your Slow Cooker.

2.   Stir and shut lid.
3.   Cook on LOW for 8 hours.
4.   Use as required !

Nutrition (Per Serving)

Calories: 33

Fat: 1g

Carbohydrates: 8g

Protein: 1g

Tantalizing Mushroom Gravy

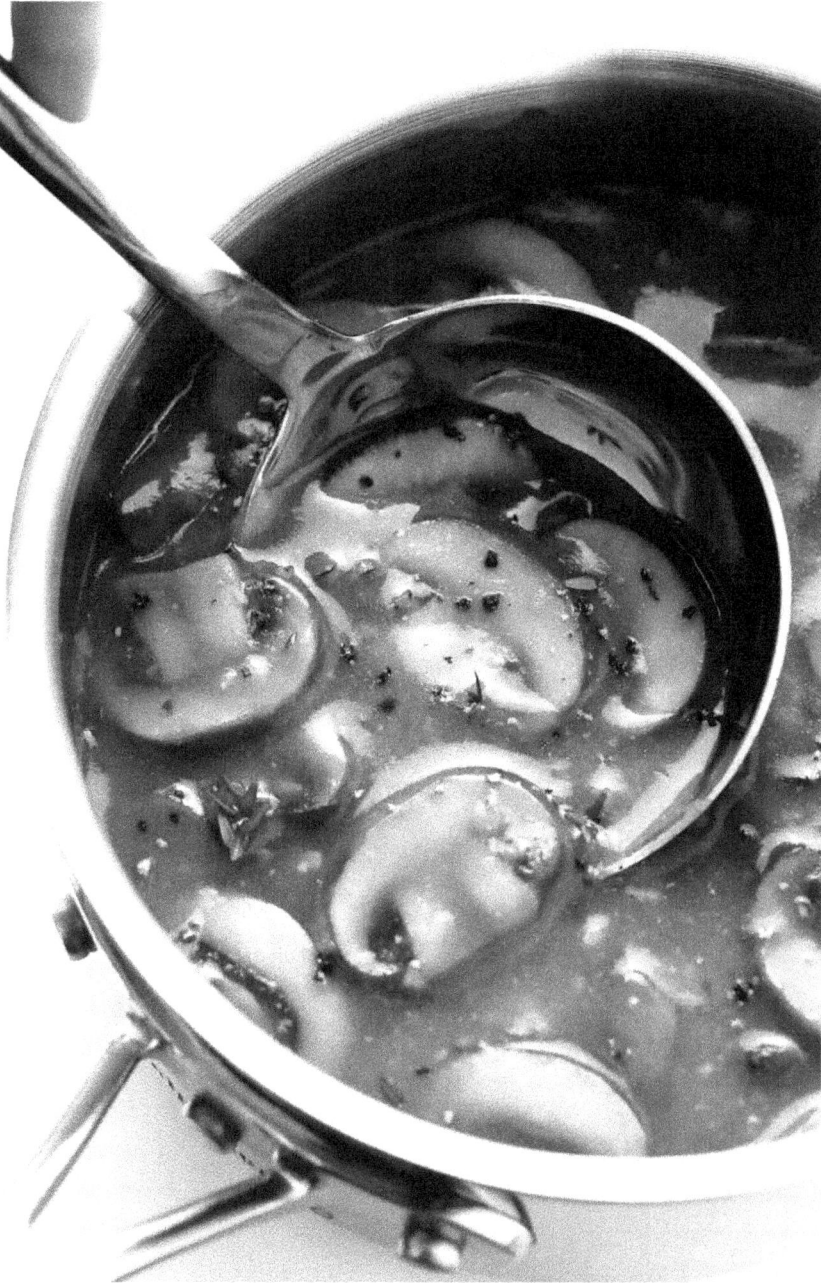

Serving: 2 cups

Prep Time: 5 minutes

Cook Time: 5-8 hours

Ingredients:

- 1 cup button mushrooms, sliced

- ¾ cup low-fat buttermilk

- 1/3 cup water

- 1 medium onion, finely diced

- 2 garlic cloves, minced

- 2 tablespoons extra virgin olive oil

- 2 tablespoons all-purpose flour
- 1 tablespoon fresh rosemary, minced Freshly ground black pepper

How To:

1. Add the listed ingredients to your Slow Cooker.

2. Place lid and cook on LOW for 5-8 hours.
3. Serve warm and use as needed!

Nutrition (Per Serving)

Calories: 54

Fat: 4g

Carbohydrates: 4g

Protein: 2g

Everyday Vegetable Stock

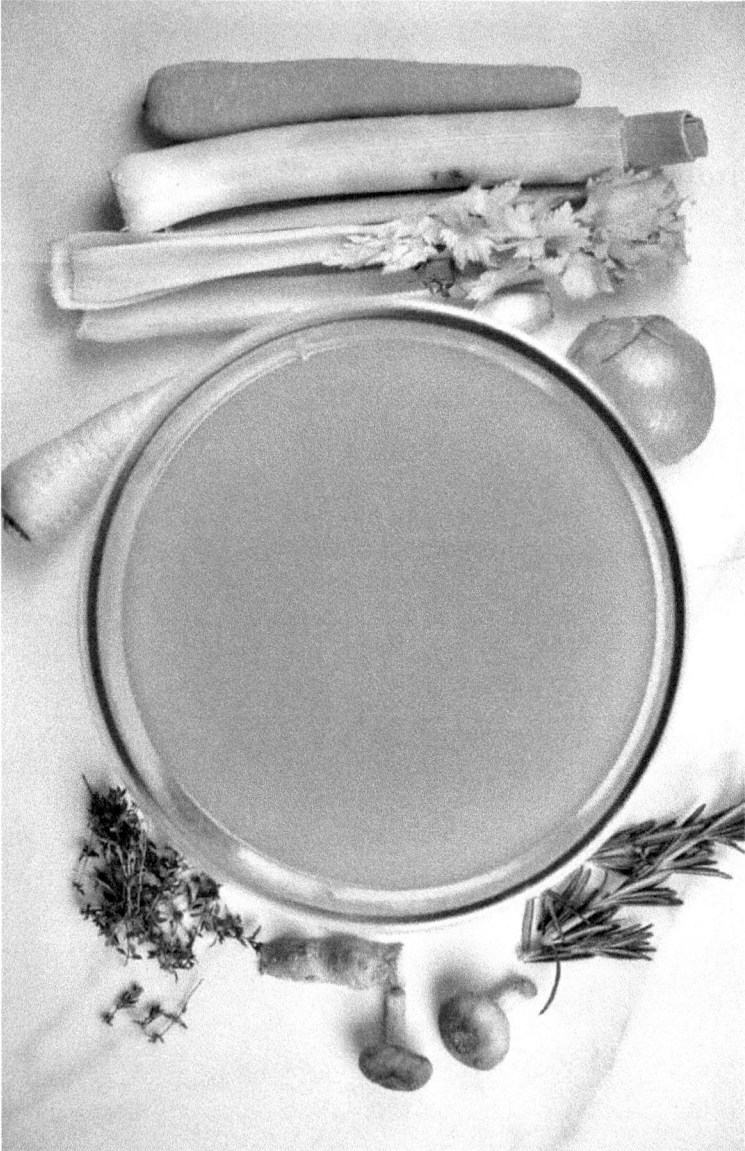

Serving: 10 cups

Prep Time: 5 minutes

Cook Time: 8-12 hours

Ingredients:

- 2 celery stalks (with leaves), quartered

- 4 ounces mushrooms, with stems

- 2 carrots, unpeeled and quartered

- 1 onion, unpeeled, quartered from pole to pole

- 1 garlic head, unpeeled, halved across middle

- 2 fresh thyme sprigs

- 10 peppercorns
- ½ teaspoon salt

- Enough water to fill 3 quarters of Slow Cooker

How To:

1. Add celery, mushrooms, onion, carrots, garlic, thyme, salt, peppercorn and water to your Slow Cooker.

2. Stir and canopy .
3. Cook on LOW for 8-12 hours.
4. Strain the stock through a fine mesh cloth/metal mesh and discard solids.
5. Use as needed.

Nutrition (Per Serving)

Calories: 38

Fat: 5g

Carbohydrates: 1g

Protein: 0g

Grilled Chicken with Lemon and Fennel

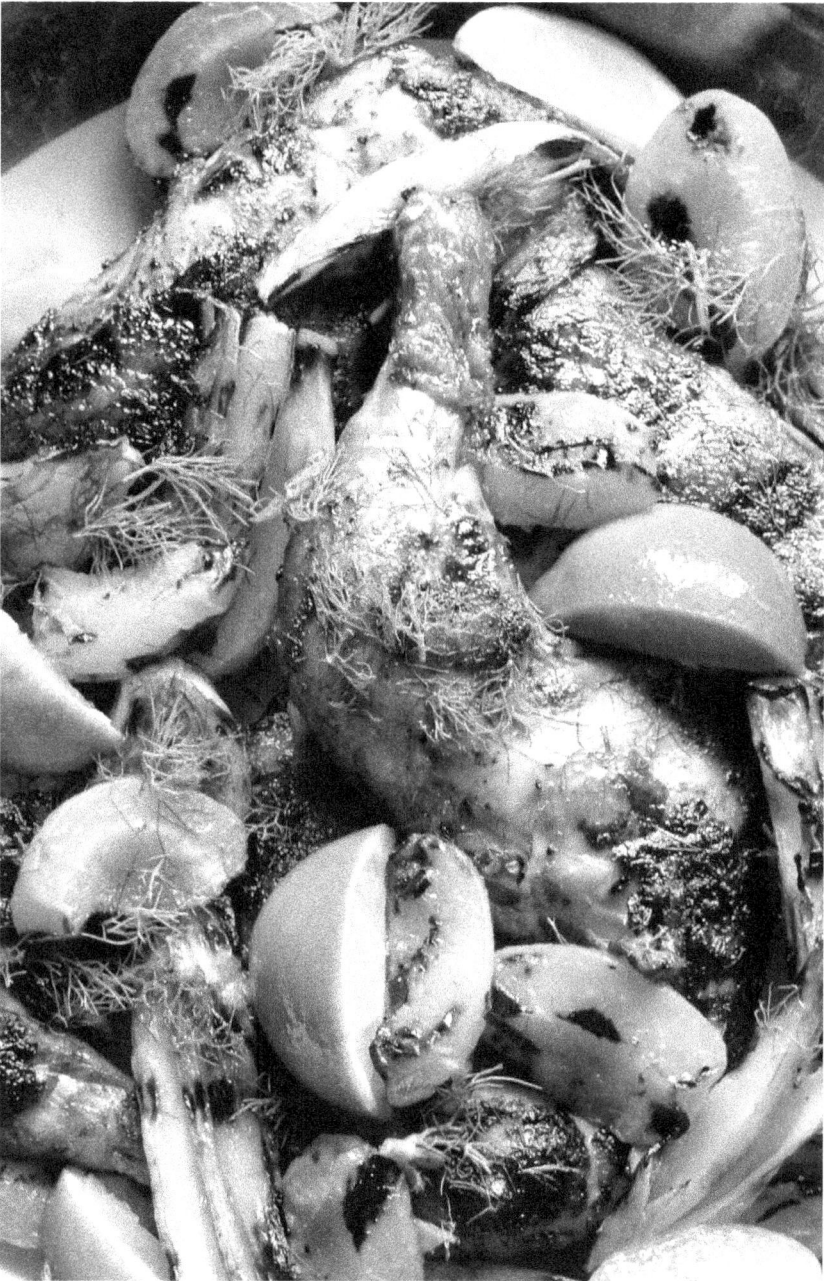

Serving: 4

Prep Time: 5 minutes

Cook Time: 25 minutes

Ingredients:

- 2 cups chicken fillets , cut and skewed

- 1 large fennel bulb

- 2 garlic cloves

- 1 jar green olives

- 1 lemon

How To:

1. Pre-heat your grill to medium-high.
2. Crush garlic cloves.

3.   Take a bowl and add vegetable oil and season with sunflower seeds and pepper.

4.   Coat chicken skewers with the marinade.

5.   Transfer them under the grill and grill for 20 minutes, ensuring to show them halfway through until golden.

6.   Zest half the lemon and cut the opposite half into quarters.

7.   Cut the fennel bulb into similarly sized segments.

8.   Brush vegetable oil everywhere the clove segments and cook for 3-5 minutes.

9.   Chop them and add them to the bowl with the marinade.

10.   Add lemon peel and olives.

11.   Once the meat is prepared , serve with the vegetable mix.

12.   Enjoy!

Nutrition (Per Serving)

Calories: 649

Fat: 16g

Carbohydrates: 33g

Protein: 18g

Caramelized Pork Chops and Onion

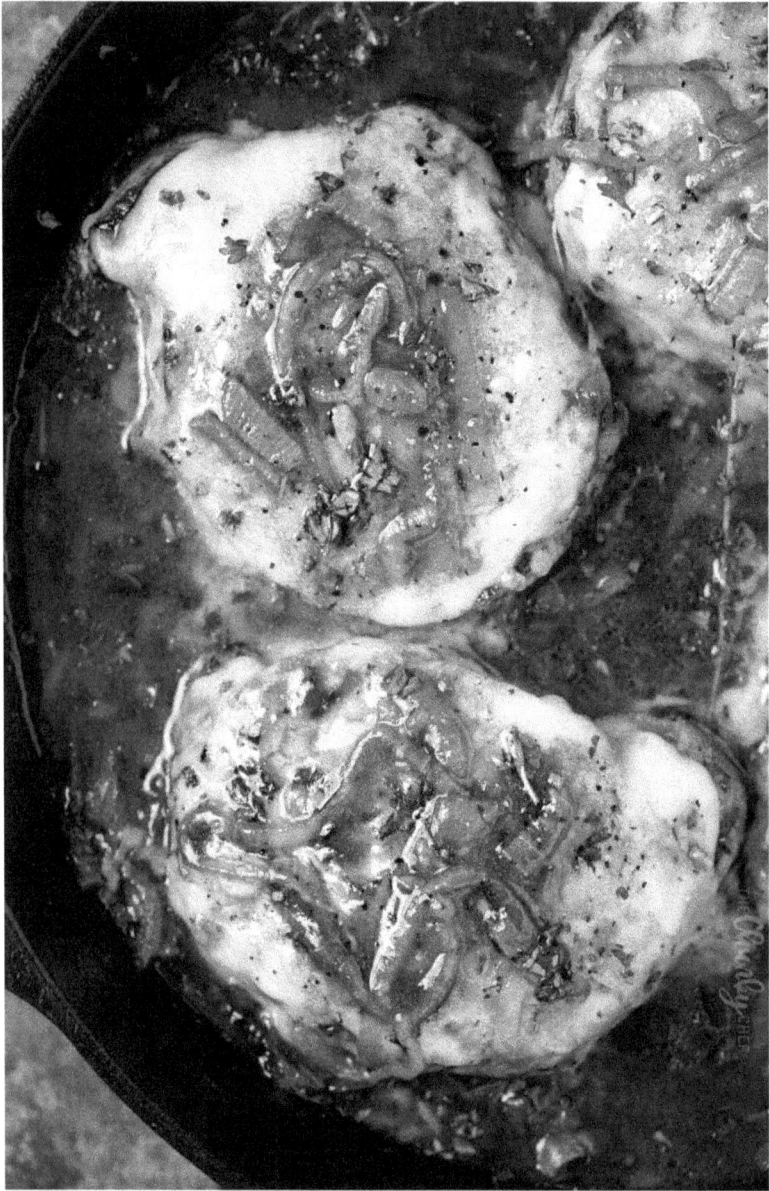

Serving: 4

Prep Time: 5 minutes

Cook Time: 40 minutes

Ingredients:

- 4-pound chuck roast

- 4 ounces green Chili, chopped

- 2 tablespoons of chili powder

- ½ teaspoon of dried oregano

- ½ teaspoon of cumin, ground

- 2 garlic cloves, minced

How To:

1.   Rub the chops with a seasoning of 1 teaspoon of pepper and a couple of teaspoons of sunflower seeds.

2. Take a skillet and place it over medium heat, add oil and permit the oil to heat up

3. Brown the seasoned chop each side .

4. Add water and onion to the skillet and canopy , lower the warmth to low and simmer for 20 minutes.

5. Turn the chops over and season with more sunflower seeds and pepper.

6. Cover and cook until the water fully evaporates and therefore the beer [MOU1]shows a rather brown texture.

7. Remove the chops and serve with a topping of the caramelized onion.

8. Serve and enjoy!

Nutrition (Per Serving)

Calorie: 47

Fat: 4g

Carbohydrates: 4g

Protein: 0.5g

Hearty Pork Belly Casserole

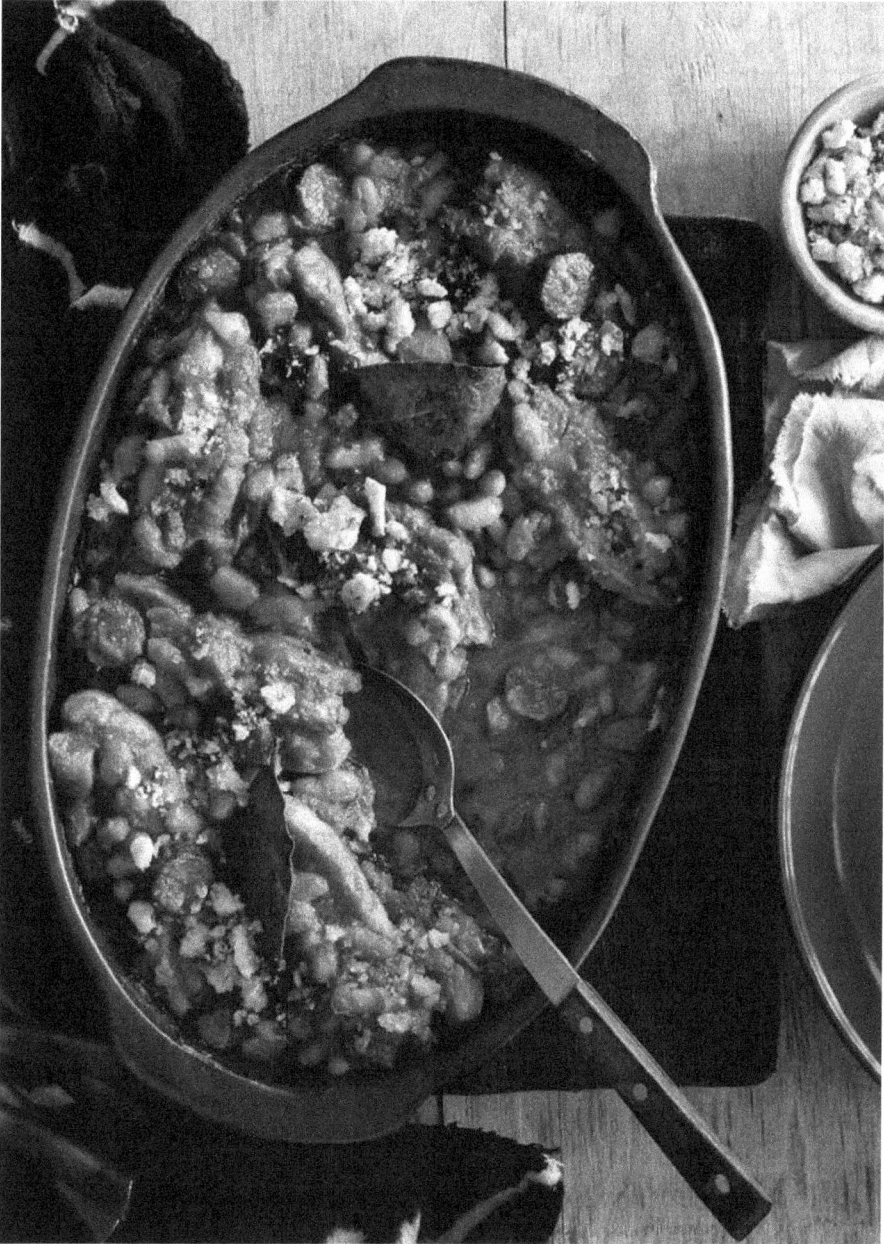

Serving: 4

Prep Time: 5 minutes

Cook Time: 25 minutes

Ingredients:

- 8 pork belly slices, cut into small pieces

- 3 large onions, chopped

- 4 tablespoons lemon

- Juice of 1 lemon

- Seasoning as you needed

How To:

1. Take an outsized autoclave and place it over medium heat.
2. Add onions and sweat them for five minutes.

3. Add side of pork slices and cook until the meat browns and onions become golden.

4. Cover with water and add honey, lemon peel , sunflower seeds, pepper, and shut the pressure seal.

5. Pressure cook for 40 minutes.

6. Serve and luxuriate in with a garnish of fresh chopped parsley if you favor .

Nutrition (Per Serving)

Calories: 753

Fat: 41g

Carbohydrates: 68g

Protein: 30g

Apple Pie Crackers

Serving: 100 crackers

Prep Time: 10 minutes

Cooking Time: 120 minutes

Ingredients:

- 2 tablespoons + 2 teaspoons avocado oil

- 1 medium Granny Smith apple, roughly chopped ¼ cup Erythritol

- 1/4 cup sunflower seeds, ground

- 1 ¾ cups roughly ground flax seeds

- 1/8 teaspoon Ground cloves

- 1/8 teaspoon ground cardamom

- 3 tablespoons nutmeg

- ¼ teaspoon ground ginger

How To:

1.   Pre-heat your oven to 225 degrees F.

2.   Line two baking sheets with parchment paper and keep them on the side.

3.   Add oil, apple, Erythritol to a bowl and blend .

4.   Transfer to kitchen appliance and add remaining ingredients, process until combined.

5.   Transfer batter to baking sheets, spread evenly and dig crackers.

6.   Bake for 1 hour, flip and bake for an additional hour.

7.   allow them to cool and serve.

8.   Enjoy!

Nutrition (Per Serving)

Total Carbs: 0.9g (%)

Fiber: 0.5g

Protein: 0.4g (%)

Fat: 2.1g (%)

Paprika Lamb Chops

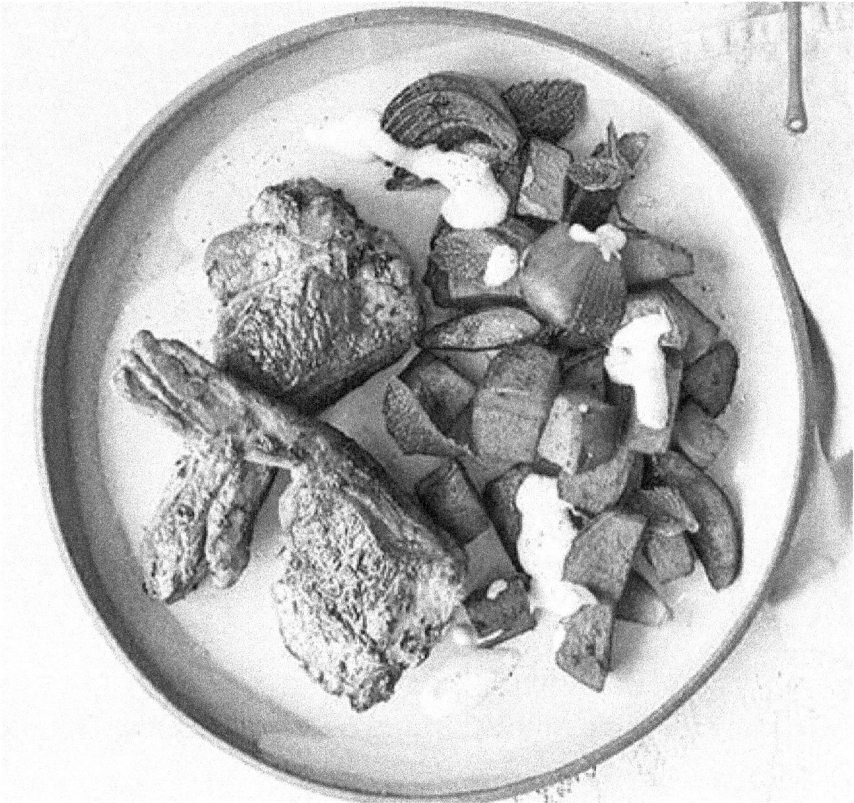

Serving: 4

Prep Time: 10 minutes

Cook Time: 15 minutes

Ingredients:

- 1 lamb rack, cut into chops pepper to taste 1 tablespoon paprika
- 1/2 cup cumin powder
- 1/2 teaspoon chili powder

How To:

1.   Take a bowl and add paprika, cumin, chili, pepper, and stir.

2.   Add lamb chops and rub the mixture.

3.   Heat grill over medium-temperature and add lamb chops, cook for five minutes.

4.   Flip and cook for five minutes more, flip again.

5.   Cook for two minutes, flip and cook for two minutes more.

6.   Serve and enjoy!

Nutrition (Per Serving)

Calories: 200

Fat: 5g

Carbohydrates: 4g

Protein: 8g

Chicken & Goat Cheese Skillet

Ingredients

- 1/2 pound of boneless skinless chicken breasts, cut into 1-inch pieces

- 1/4 teaspoon salt

- 1/8 teaspoon pepper

- Two teaspoons olive oil

- 1 cup sliced fresh asparagus (1-inch pieces)

- One garlic clove, minced

- Three plum tomatoes, chopped

- Three tablespoons 2% milk

- Two tablespoons herbed fresh goat cheese, crumbled Hot cooked rice or pasta

- Additional goat cheese, optional

Directions

1. Toss chicken with salt and pepper. Heat oil at medium heat; saute chicken until not pink, 4-6 minutes.Remove from pan; keep warm.

2. Add asparagus to skillet; cook and blend at medium-high heat 1 minute. Add garlic; cook and stir 30 seconds. Stirin tomatoes, milk, and two tablespoons cheese; cook, covered, over medium heat until cheese begins to melt, 2-3 minutes. Stir in chicken. Serve with rice. If desired, top with additional cheese.

Nutrition

251 calories, 11g fat, 74mg cholesterol, 447mg sodium, 8g carbohydrate (5g sugars, 3g fiber), 29g protein. Diabetic Exchanges: 4 lean meat, two fat, one vegetable.

Green Curry Salmon with Green Beans

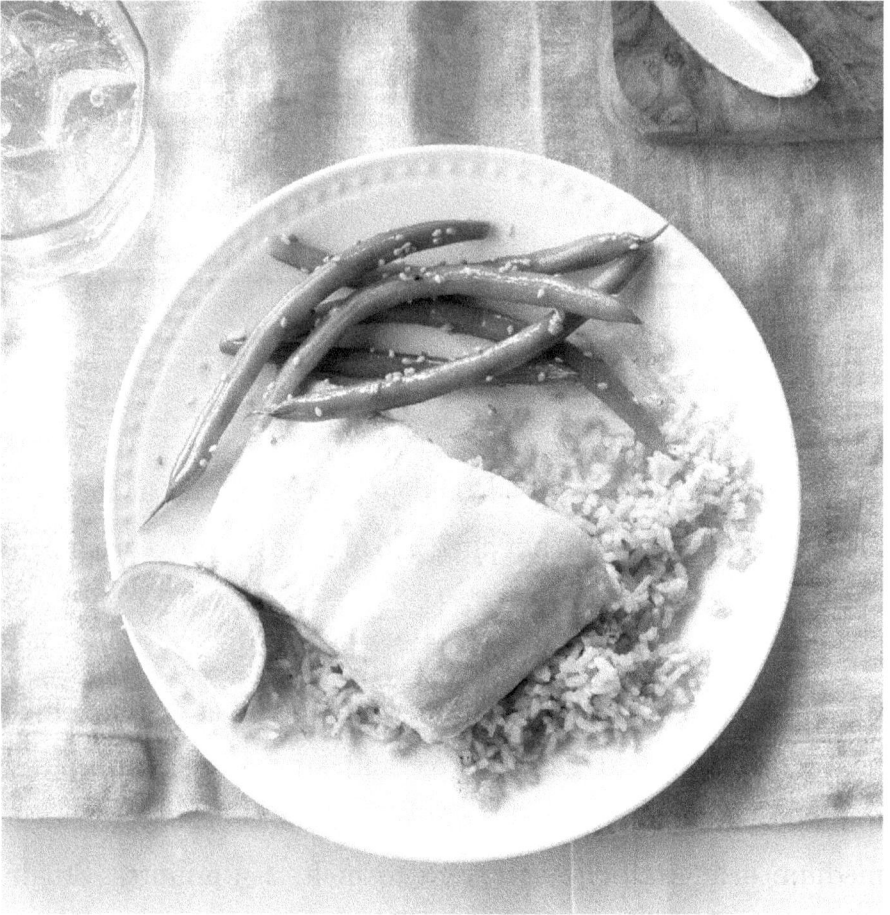

Ingredients

- Four salmon fillets (4 ounces each)

- 1 cup light coconut milk

- Two tablespoons green curry paste

- 1 cup uncooked instant brown rice

- 1 cup reduced-sodium chicken broth

- 1/8 teaspoon pepper

- 3/4 pound fresh green beans, trimmed

- One teaspoon sesame oil

- One teaspoon sesame seeds, toasted

- Lime wedges

Directions

1.   Preheat oven to 400°. Place salmon in an 8-in. Square baking dish. Mix together coconut milk and curry paste; pour over salmon. Bake, uncovered, till fish simply starts offevolved to flake effortlessly with a fork, 15-20 minutes.

2.   Meanwhile, during a small saucepan, integrate rice, broth and pepper; convey to a boil. Reduce warmth; simmer, covered, 5 minutes. Remove from heat; let stand five minutes.

3.   In a big saucepan, area steamer basket over 1 in. Of water. Place inexperienced beans inside the basket; convey water to a boil. Reduce heat to take care of a simmer; steam, covered, till beans are crisp-tender, 7-10 minutes. Toss with vegetable oil and sesame seeds.

4.   Serve salmon with rice, beans and lime wedges. Spoon coconut sauce over the salmon.

Nutrition Facts

366 calories, 17g fat (5g saturated fat), 57mg cholesterol, 340mg sodium, 29g carbohydrate (5g sugars, 4g fibre), 24g protein.

Chicken Veggie Packets

Ingredients

- Four boneless and skinless chicken breast halves (4 ounces each) 1/2 pound sliced fresh mushrooms 1-1/2 cups fresh baby carrots

- 1 cup pearl onions

- 1/2 cup julienned sweet red pepper

- 1/4 teaspoon pepper

- Three teaspoons minced fresh thyme

- 1/2 teaspoon salt, optional

- Lemon wedges, optional

Directions

1.   Flatten bird breasts to 1/2-in. Thickness; vicinity every on a touch of industrial quality foil (about 12 in. Square). Layer the mushrooms, carrots, onions and pink pepper over bird; sprinkle with pepper, thyme and salt if desired.

2.   Fold foil around hen and greens and seal tightly. Place on a baking sheet. Bake at 375° for a half-hour or until chook juices run clear. If desired, serve with lemon wedges.

Nutrition Facts

175 calories, 3g fat (1g saturated fat), 63mg cholesterol, 100mg sodium, 11g carbohydrate (6g sugars, 2g fibre), 25g protein.

Sweet Onion & Sausage Spaghetti

Ingredients

- 6 ounces uncooked whole-wheat spaghetti

- 3/4 pound Italian turkey sausage links, casings removed
  Two teaspoons olive oil

- One sweet onion, thinly sliced

- 1-pint cherry tomatoes halved

- One and a half cup of fresh basil leaves (sliced)

- 1/2 cup half-and-half cream

- Shaved Parmesan cheese, optional

Directions

1.   Cook spaghetti consistent with directions given. At an equivalent time, during a large nonstick skillet over medium heat, cook sausage in oil for five minutes. Add onion; bake 8-10 minutes

longer or until meat is not any longer pink and onion is tender.

2.   Stir in tomatoes and basil; heat through. Add cream; bring back a boil. Drain spaghetti; toss with sausage mixture. Garnish with cheese if desired.

Nutrition Facts

334 calories, 12g fat (4g saturated fat), 46mg cholesterol, 378mg sodium, 41g carbohydrate (8g sugars, 6g fibre), 17g protein.

Beef and Blue Cheese Penne with Pesto

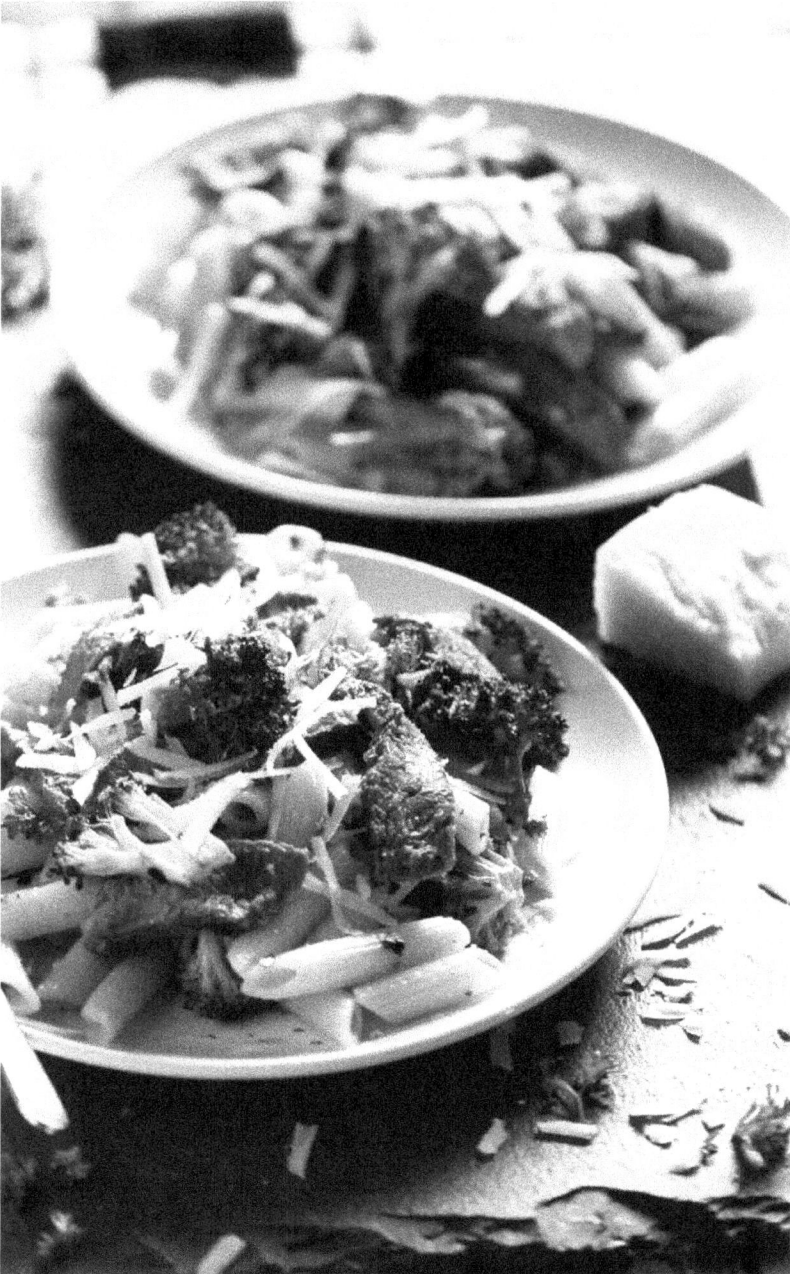

Ingredients

- 2 cups uncooked whole wheat penne pasta

- Two beef tenderloin steaks (6 ounces each)

- 1/4 teaspoon salt

- 1/4 teaspoon pepper

- 5 ounces of fresh baby spinach (about 6 cups), coarsely chopped

- 2 cups grape tomatoes, halved

- 1/3 cup prepared pesto

- 1/4 cup chopped walnuts

- 1/4 cup crumbled Gorgonzola cheese

Directions

1.   Cook pasta consistent with package directions.

2.   Meanwhile, sprinkle steaks with salt and pepper. Grill steaks, covered, over medium heat. Heat for 5-7 mins on all sides or until meat reaches desired doneness.

3.   Drain pasta; transfer to an outsized bowl. Add spinach, tomatoes, pesto and walnuts; toss to coat. Cut steak into thin slices. Serve pasta mixture with beef; sprinkle with cheese.

Nutrition Facts

532 calories, 22g fat (6g saturated fat), 50mg cholesterol, 434mg sodium, 49g carbohydrate (3g sugars, 9g fibre), 35g protein.

Asparagus Turkey Stir-Fry

Ingredients

- Two teaspoons cornstarch

- 1/4 cup chicken broth

- One tablespoon lemon juice

- One teaspoon soy sauce

- 1 pound of turkey breast tenderloins, cut into 1/2-inch strips One garlic clove, minced

- Two tablespoons canola oil, divided

- 1 pound of asparagus, cut into 1-1/2-inch pieces One jar (2 ounces) sliced pimientos, drained

Instructions

1.   In a little bowl, mix the cornstarch, broth, juice and soy until smooth; put aside . during a large skillet orwok, stir-fry turkey and garlic in 1 tablespoon oil until meat is not any longer pink; remove and keep warm.

2.   Stir-fry asparagus in remaining oil until crisp-tender. Add pimientos. Stir the mixture and increase the pan; cook andstir for 1 minute or until thickened. Return turkey to the pan; heat through.

Nutrition Facts

205 calories, 9g fat (1g saturated fat), 56mg cholesterol, 204mg sodium, 5g carbohydrate (1g sugars, 1g fibre), 28g protein.

Chicken with Celery Root Puree

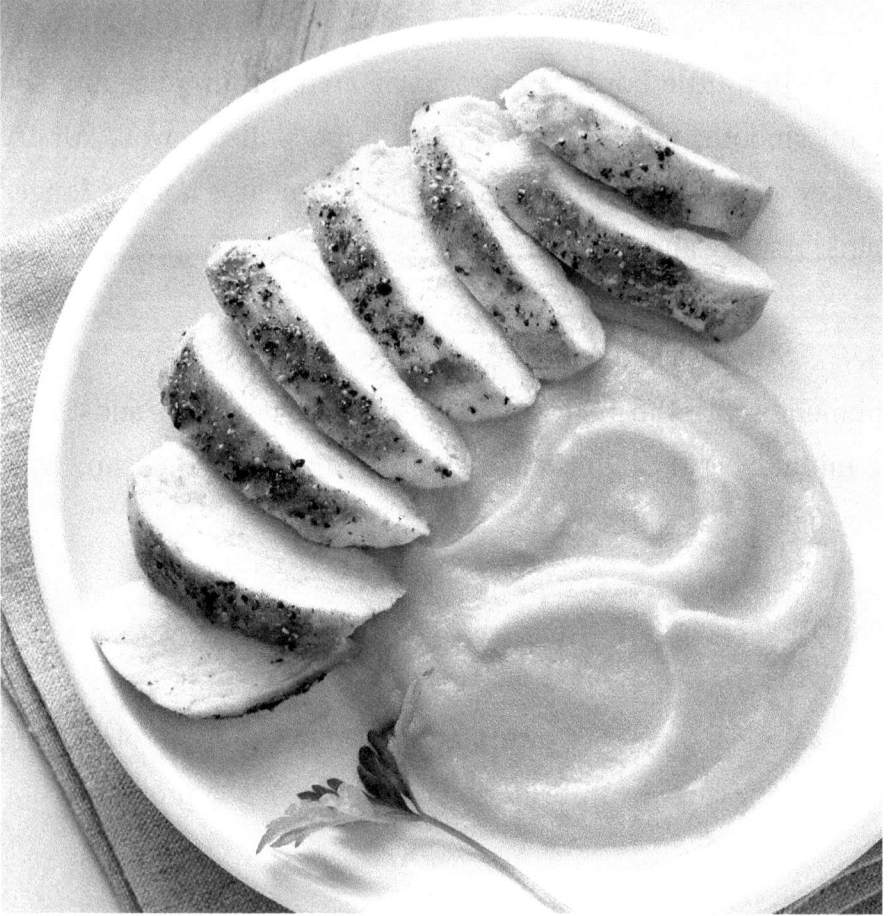

Ingredients

- Four boneless skinless chicken breast halves (6 ounces each)

- 1/2 teaspoon pepper

- 1/4 teaspoon salt

- Three teaspoons canola oil, divided

- One large celery root, peeled and chopped (about 3 cups)

- 2 cups diced peeled butternut squash

- One small onion, chopped

- Two garlic cloves, minced

- 2/3 cup unsweetened apple juice

Instructions

1.   Sprinkle chicken with pepper and salt. Take an outsized skillet and coat with cooking spray, heat two teaspoons oil over

medium heat. Brown chicken on each side . Remove chicken from pan.

2.   Heat the remaining oil over medium-high within the same pan. Add celery root, squash and onion; cook and stir until squash is crisp-tender. Add garlic; cook 1 minute longer.

3.   Return chicken to pan; add fruit juice . bring back a boil. Reduce heat; simmer, covered, 12-15 minutes or until a thermometer inserted in chicken reads 165°.

4.   Remove chicken; keep warm. Cool vegetable mixture slightly. Process during a kitchen appliance until smooth. Return to pan and warmth through. Serve with chicken.

Nutrition Facts

328 calories, 8g fat (1g saturated fat), 94mg cholesterol, 348mg sodium, 28g carbohydrate (10g sugars, 5g fibre), 37g protein.

Apple-Cherry Pork Medallions

Ingredients

- One pork tenderloin (1 pound)

- One teaspoon minced fresh rosemary or 1/4 teaspoon dried rosemary, crushed

- One teaspoon minced fresh thyme or 1/4 teaspoon dried thyme

- 1/2 teaspoon celery salt

- One tablespoon olive oil

- One large apple, sliced

- 2/3 cup unsweetened apple juice

- Three tablespoons dried tart cherries

- One tablespoon honey

- One tablespoon cider vinegar

- One package (8.8 ounces) ready-to-serve brown rice

Instructions

1. Cut tenderloin crosswise into 12 slices; sprinkle with rosemary, thyme and flavorer . during a huge skillet, heat oil over medium-excessive heat. Brown pork on both sides; do away with from pan.

2.   In the equal skillet, combine apple, fruit juice , cherries, honey and vinegar. Boil it and stirring to loosen browned bits from pan. Reduce warmness; simmer, uncovered, 3-four minutes or simply till apple is tender.

3.   Return meat to the pan, turning to coat with sauce; cook, covered, 3-4 minutes or till meat is tender. Meanwhile, put together rice keep with package deal directions; serve with meat mixture.

Nutrition Facts

349 calories, 9g fat (2g saturated fat), 64mg cholesterol, 179mg sodium, 37g carbohydrate (16g sugars, 4g fibre), and 25g protein.

Butternut Turkey Soup

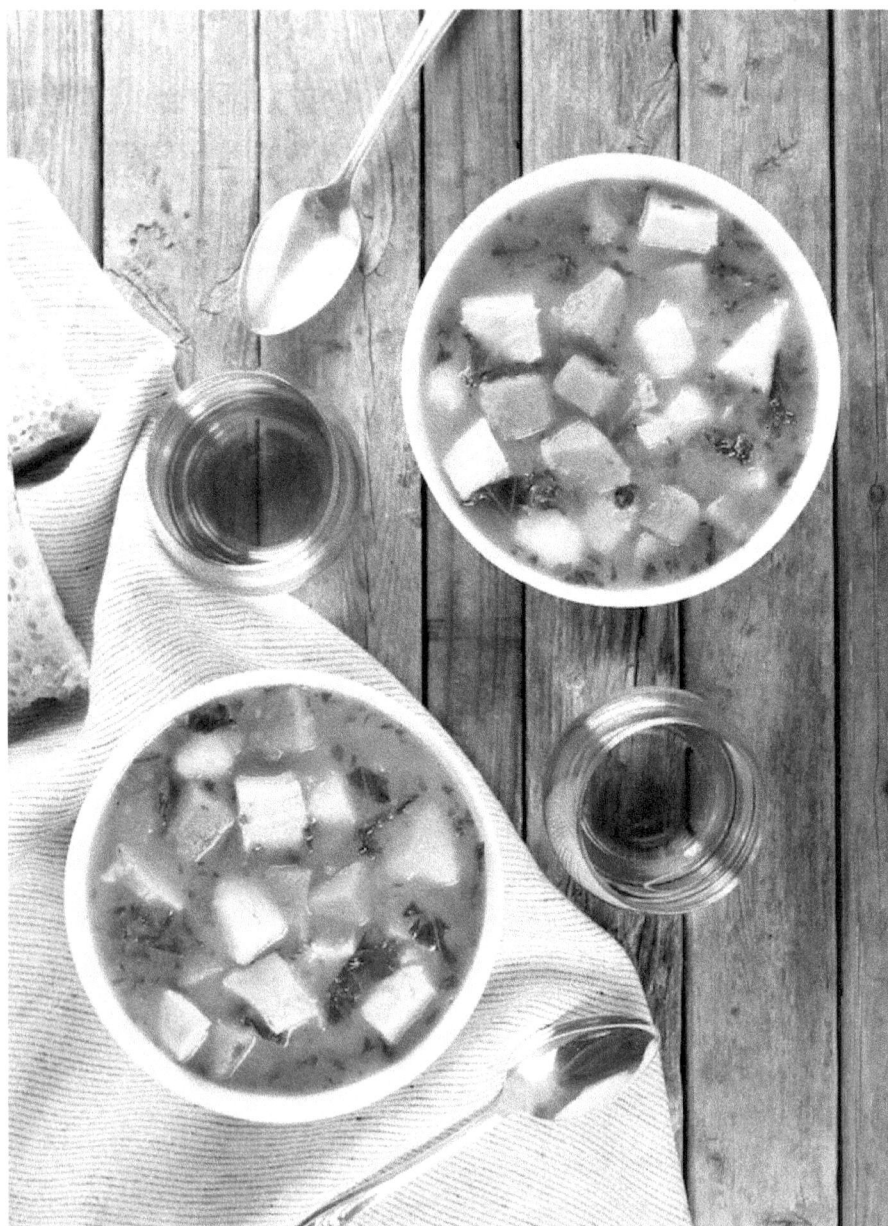

Ingredients

- Three shallots, thinly sliced

- One tsp of olive oil

- 3 cups of reduced-sodium chicken broth

- 3 cups of cubed peeled butternut squash (3/4-inch cubes) Two medium-sized red potatoes, cut into 1/2-inch cubes 1-1/2 cups of water

- Two teaspoons of minced fresh thyme

- 1/2 teaspoon pepper

- Two whole cloves

- 3 cups cubed cooked turkey breast

Instructions

1.   In a large-size saucepan coated with cooking spray, cook dinner shallots in oil over medium heat till tender. Stir within the broth, squash, potatoes, water, thyme and pepper.

2.   Place spices on a double thickness of cheesecloth; carry up corners of the material and tie with string to shape a bag. Stir into soup. bring back a boil. Reduce warmness; cowl and simmer for 10-15 mins or till vegetables are tender. Stir in turkey; warmth through. Discard spice bag.

Nutrition

192 calories, 2g fat (0 saturated fat), 60mg cholesterol, 332mg sodium, 20g carbohydrate (3g sugars, 3g fibre), 25g protein.

Black Bean & Sweet Potato Rice Bowls

Ingredients

- 3/4 cup uncooked long-grain rice

- 1/4 teaspoon garlic salt

- 1-1/2 cups water

- Three tablespoons olive oil, divided

- One large sweet potato, peeled and diced

- One medium red onion, finely chopped

- 4 cups chopped fresh kale (sturdy stems removed) One can (15 ounces) black beans, rinsed and drained Two tablespoons sweet chilli sauce Lime wedges, optional

- Additional sweet chilli sauce, optional

Instructions

1.   Place rice, flavorer and water during a large saucepan; bring back a boil. Reduce heat; simmer, covered until liquid is absorbed and rice is tender 15-20 minutes. Remove from heat; let stand 5 minutes.

2.   At an equivalent time take an outsized pan and warmth two tablespoons oil over medium-high heat; saute sweet potato 8 minutes. Add onion; cook and stir until potato is tender 4-6 minutes. Add kale; cook and stir until tender, 3-5 minutes. Stir in beans; heat through.

3.   Gently stir two tablespoons chilli sauce and remaining oil into rice; increase potato mixture. If you would like , serve with lime wedges and extra chilli sauce.

Nutrition

435 calories, 11g fat (2g saturated fat), 0 cholesterol, 405mg sodium, 74g carbohydrate (15g sugars, 8g fibre), 10g protein.

Pepper Ricotta Primavera

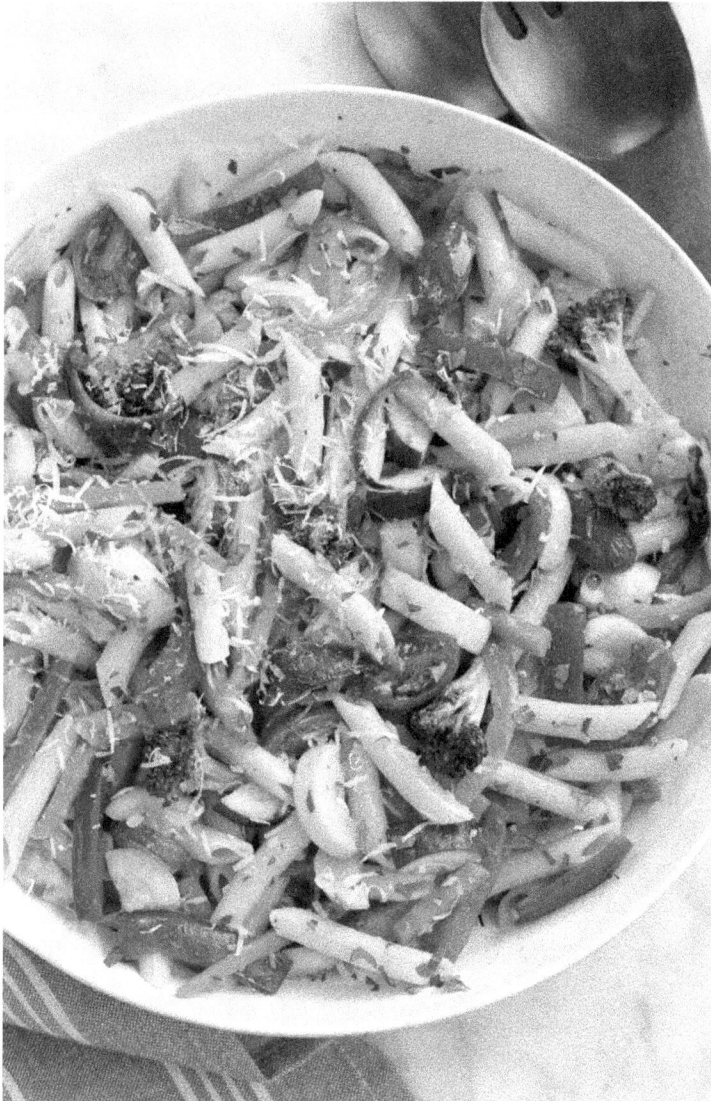

Ingredients

- 1 cup part-skim ricotta cheese

- 1/2 cup fat-free milk

- Four teaspoons olive oil

- One garlic clove, minced

- 1/2 teaspoon crushed red pepper flakes One medium green pepper, julienned One medium sweet red pepper, julienned One medium fresh yellow pepper, julienned One medium zucchini, sliced 1 cup frozen peas, thawed

- 1/4 teaspoon dried oregano

- 1/4 teaspoon dried basil

- 6 ounces fettuccine, cooked and drained

Instructions

1.   Whisk together ricotta cheese and milk; put aside . Take an outsized skillet, heat oil over medium heat. Add garlic and pepper; saute 1 minute. Add subsequent seven ingredients. Cook and blend over medium heat until vegetables are crisptender, about 5 minutes.

2.   Add cheese mixture to fettuccine; top with vegetables. Toss to coat. Serve immediately.

Nutrition

229 calories, 7g fat (3g saturated fat), 13mg cholesterol, 88mg sodium, 31g carbohydrate (6g sugars, 4g fibre), 11g protein.

Bow Ties with Sausage & Asparagus

Ingredients

- 3 cups of uncooked whole wheat bow tie pasta (about 8 ounces)

- 1 pound of asparagus, cut into 1-1/2-inch pieces

- One package (19-1/2 ounces) Italian turkey sausage links, casings removed

- One medium onion, chopped

- Three garlic cloves, minced

- 1/4 cup shredded Parmesan cheese

- Additional shredded Parmesan cheese, optional

Instructions

1.   In a 6-qt. Stockpot, prepare dinner pasta in line with package directions, including asparagus over the last 2-three minutes of cooking. Drain, reserving half cup pasta water; return pasta and asparagus to the pot.

2.   Meanwhile, during a big skillet, cook sausage, onion and garlic over medium heat until no pink, 6-8 minutes, breaking sausage into large crumbles. increase stockpot. Stir in 1/four cup cheese and reserved pasta water as desired. Serve with additional cheese if desired.

Nutrition

247 calories, 7g fat (2g saturated fat), 36mg cholesterol, 441mg sodium, 28g carbohydrate (2g sugars, 4g fibre), 17g protein

Pork and Balsamic Strawberry Salad

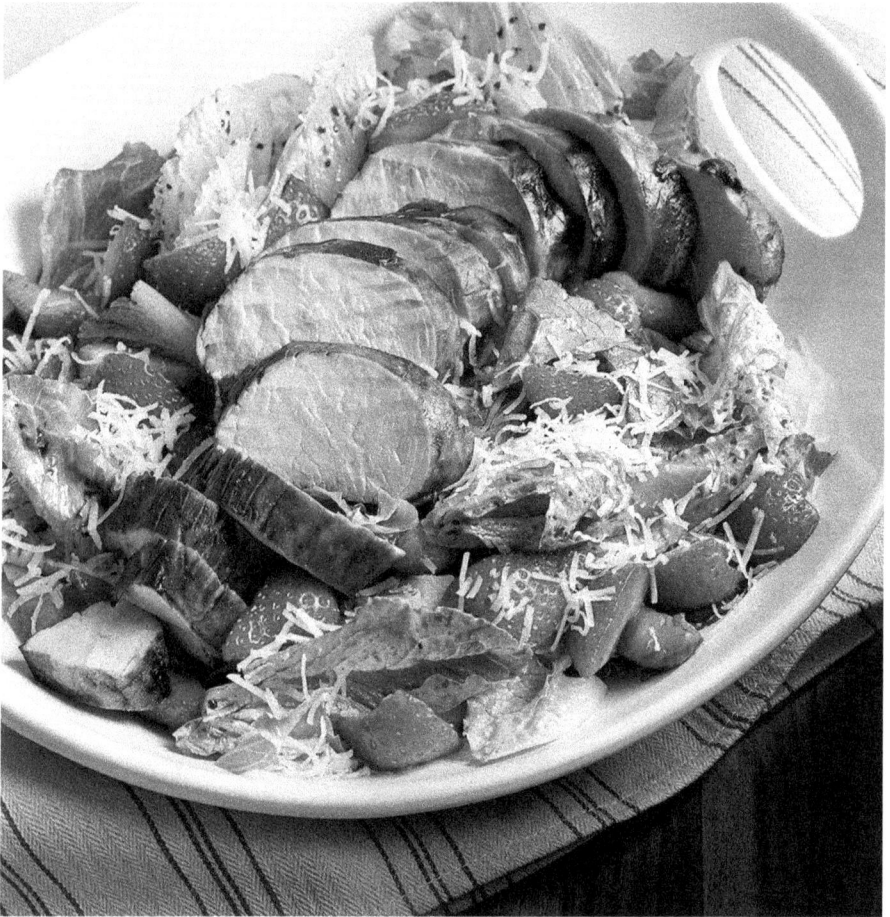

Ingredients

- One pork tenderloin (1 pound)

- 1/2 cup Italian salad dressing

- 1-1/2 cups halved fresh strawberries

- Two tablespoons balsamic vinegar

- Two teaspoons sugar

- 1/4 teaspoon salt

- 1/4 teaspoon pepper

- Two tablespoons olive oil

- 1/4 cup chicken broth

- One package about 5 ounces spring mix salad greens 1/2 cup crumbled goat cheese

Instructions

1.   Place pork during a shallow dish. Add salad dressing; flip for coating. Refrigerate and canopy for a minimum of eight hours. Mix strawberries, vinegar and sugar; cover and refrigerate.

2.   Preheat oven to 425°. Drain and wipe off meat , discarding marinade. Sprinkle with salt and pepper. during a large cast-iron or every other ovenproof skillet, warmness oil over medium-high warmness. Add beef; brown on all sides.

3.   Bake until a thermometer reads 145°, 15-20 minutes. Remove from skillet; permit or stand 5 min. Then, add broth to skillet; cook over medium warmth, stirring to loosen browned bits from pan. bring back a boil. Reduce warmth; add strawberry. Then heat it.

4.   Place green vegetables on a serving platter; sprinkle with cheese. Slice pork; found out over veggies. Top with strawberry mixture.

Nutrition

291 calories, 16g fat (5g saturated fat), 81mg cholesterol, 444mg sodium, 12g carbohydrate (7g sugars, 3g fibre), 26g protein.

Peppered Tuna Kabobs

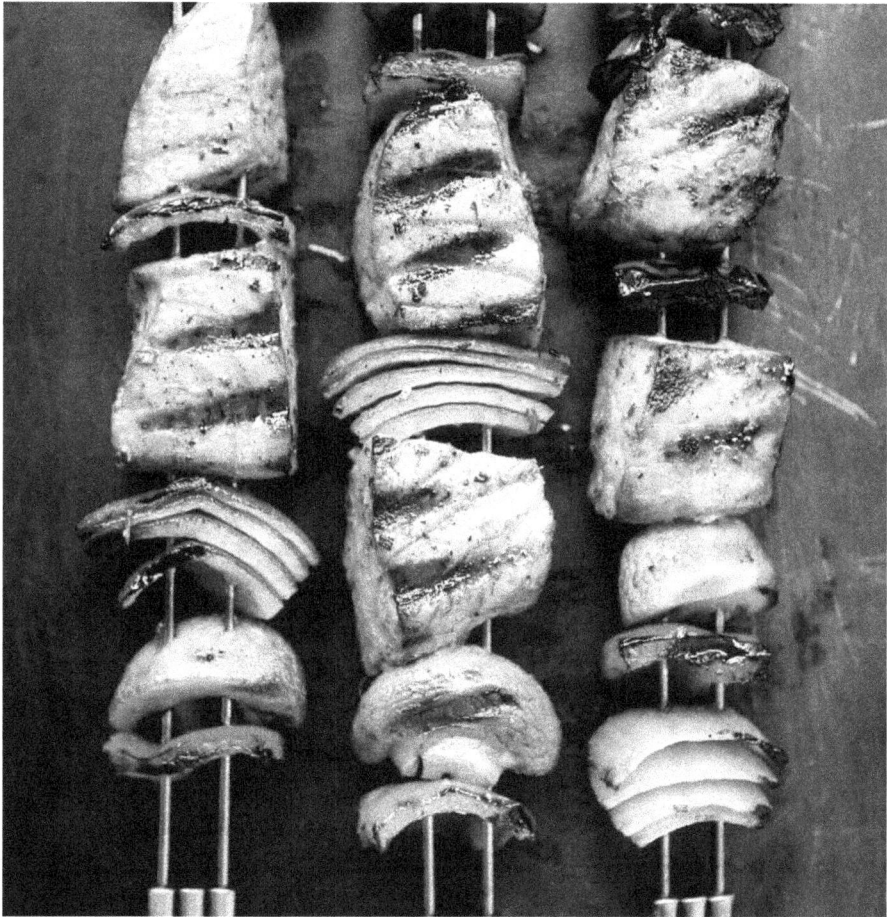

Ingredients

- 1/2 cup frozen corn, thawed Four green onions, chopped
  One jalapeno pepper, seeded and chopped

- Two tablespoons coarsely chopped fresh parsley Two tablespoons lime juice

- 1 pound tuna steaks, cut into 1-inch cubes One teaspoon coarsely ground pepper

- Two large sweet red peppers, cut into 2x1-inch pieces

Instructions

1.   One medium mango, peeled and cut into 1-inch cubes

2.   For salsa, during a small bowl, combine the primary five ingredients; put aside .

3.   Rub tuna with pepper. On 4metal or soaked wooden skewers, alternately thread red peppers, tuna and mango.

4.   Place skewers on greased grill rack. Cook, covered, over medium heat, occasionally turning, until tuna is slightly pink in centre

(medium-rare) and peppers are tender 10-12 minutes. Serve with salsa.

Nutrition

205 calories, 2g fat (0 saturated fat), 51mg cholesterol, 50mg sodium, 20g carbohydrate (12g sugars, 4g fibre), 29g protein.

Weeknight Chicken Chop Suey

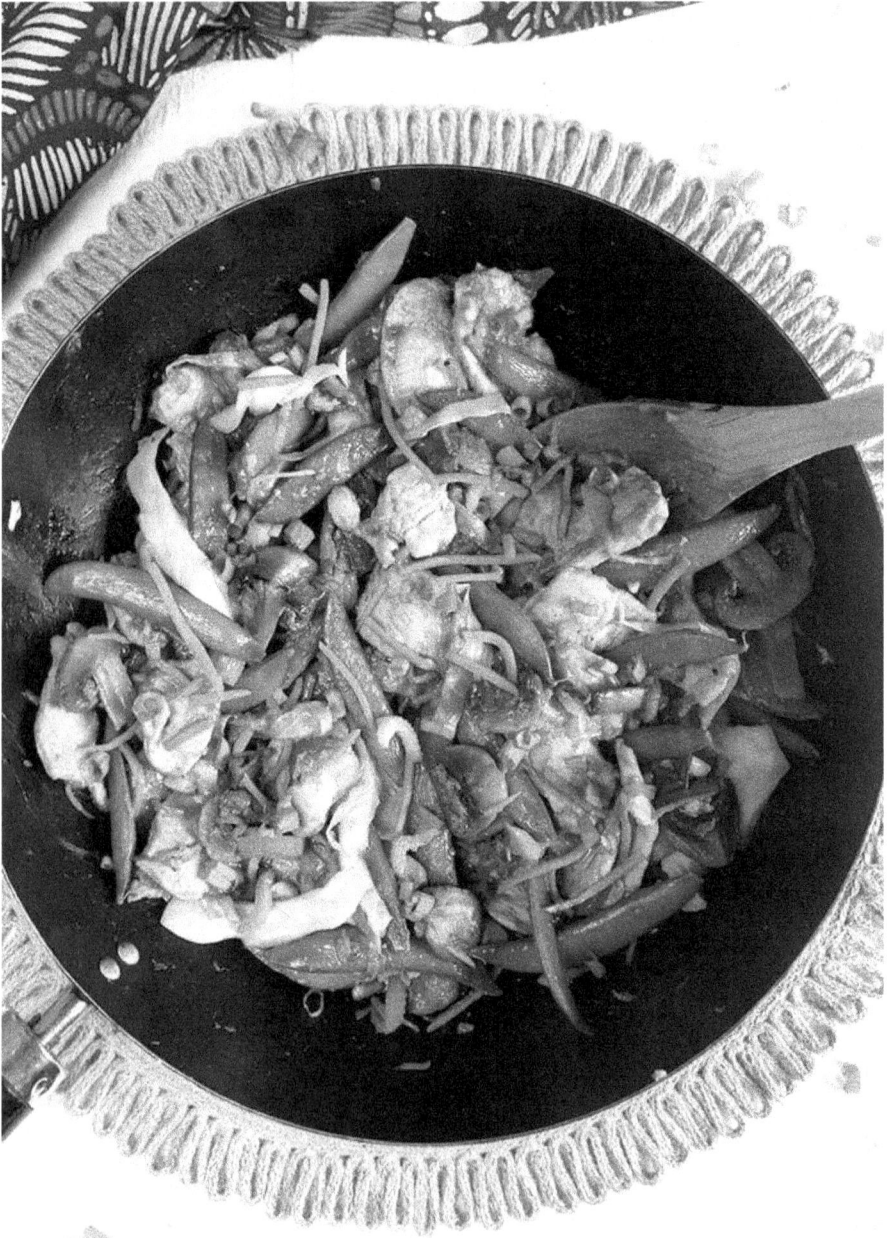

Ingredients

- Four teaspoons of olive oil

- 1 pound of boneless chicken breast side, cut into 1-inch cubes

- 1/2 teaspoon dried tarragon

- 1/2 teaspoon dried basil

- 1/2 teaspoon dried marjoram

- 1/2 teaspoon grated lemon zest

- 1-1/2 cups chopped carrots

- 1 cup unsweetened pineapple tidbits, drained (reserve juice)

- One can (8 ounces) sliced water chestnuts, drained

- One medium tart apple, chopped
- 1/2 cup chopped onion

- 1 cup cold water, divided

- Three tablespoons unsweetened pineapple juice

- Three tablespoons reduced-sodium teriyaki sauce

- Two tablespoons cornstarch

- 3 cups hot cooked brown rice

Instructions

1.   In a massive cast-iron or another heavy skillet, heat oil at medium temperature. Add chicken, herbs and lemon zest; leave it until lightly browned. Add subsequent five ingredients. Stir in

3/four cup water, fruit juice and teriyaki sauce; bring back a boil. Reduce warmness; simmer covered till chicken is not any longer purple, and therefore the carrots are gentle 10-15 minutes.

2.   Combine cornstarch and remaining water. Gradually stir into hen mixture. Leave for boiling; cook and stir till thickened, about 2 minutes. Serve with rice.

Nutrition

330 calories, 6g fat, 42mg cholesterol, 227mg sodium, 50g carbohydrate (14g sugars, 5g fibre), 20g protein

Thai Chicken Pasta Skillet

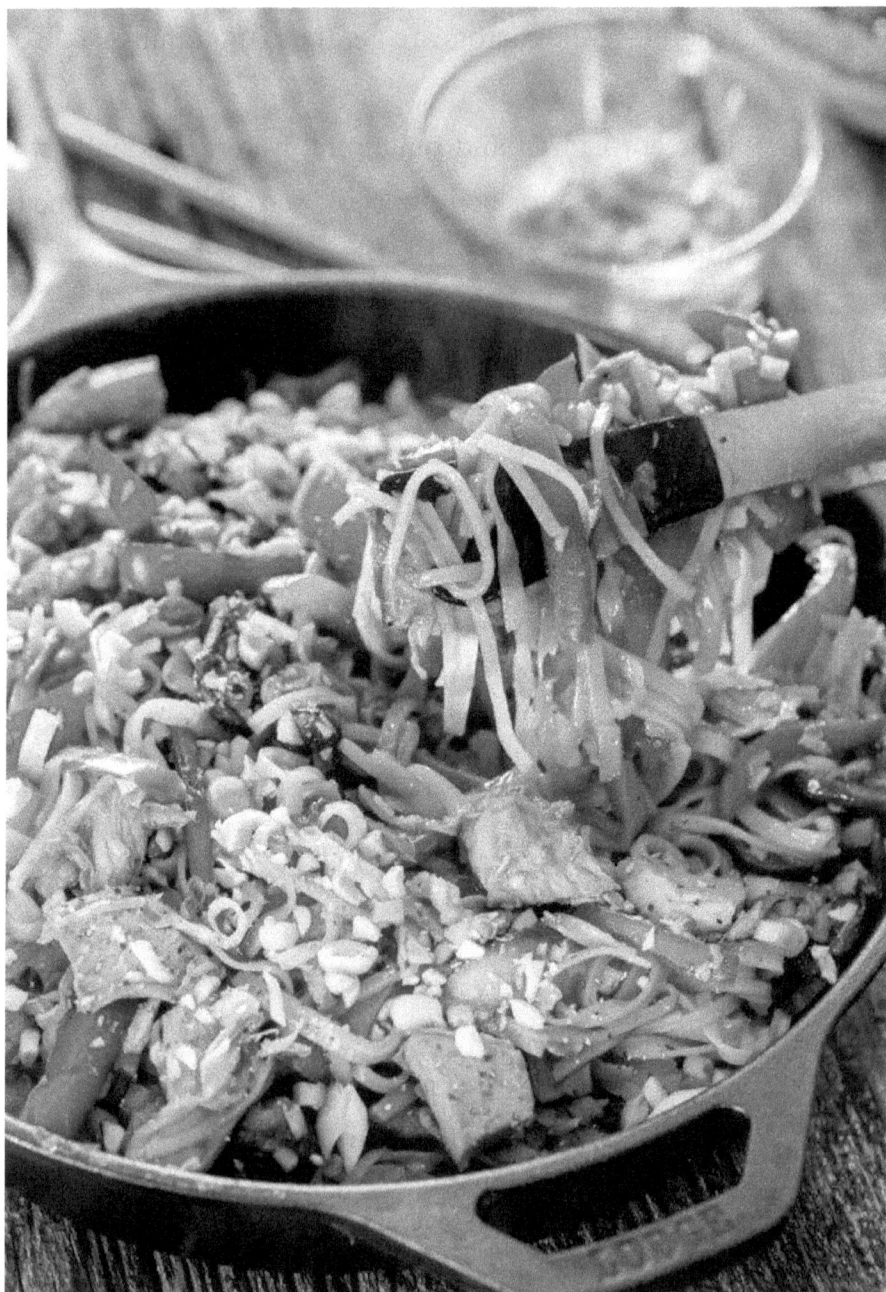

Ingredients

- 6 ounces uncooked whole-wheat spaghetti Two teaspoons canola oil

- One package (10 ounces) fresh sugar snap peas, trimmed and cut diagonally into thin strips

- 2 cups julienned carrots (about 8 ounces)

- 2 cups shredded cooked chicken

- 1 cup Thai peanut sauce

- One medium cucumber, halved lengthwise, seeded and sliced diagonally

Chopped fresh cilantro, optional
Instructions

1.   Cook spaghetti according to package directions; drain.

2.   Then, during a large skillet, heat oil a medium-high heat. Add snap peas and carrots; stir-fry 6-8 minutes or until crisptender. Add chicken, peanut sauce and spaghetti; heat through, tossing to mix .

3.   Transfer to a serving plate. Top with cucumber and, if desired, cilantro.

Nutrition Facts

403 calories, 15g fat (3g saturated fat), 42mg cholesterol, 432mg sodium, 43g carbohydrate (15g sugars, 6g fibre), 25g protein

Spinach-Orzo Salad with Chickpeas

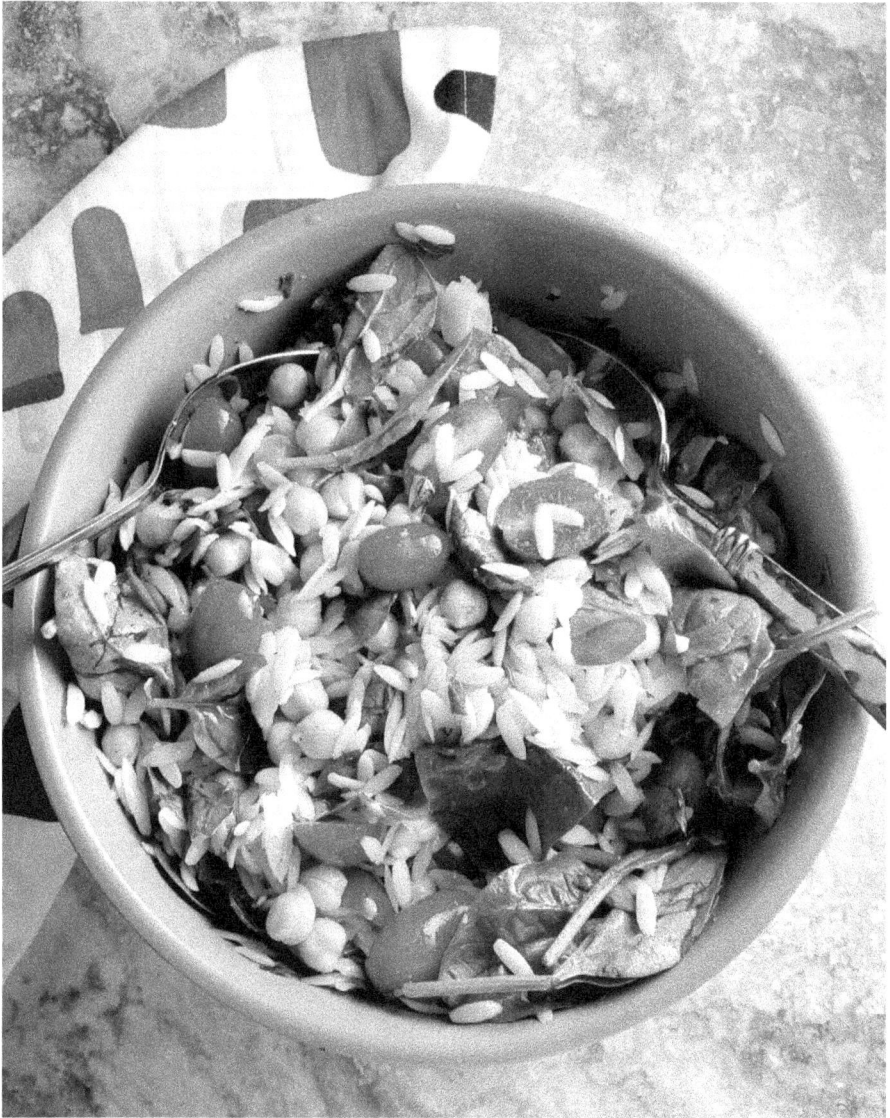

Ingredients

- One 14-1/2 ounces reduced-sodium chicken broth 1-1/2 cups of uncooked whole wheat orzo pasta 4 cups of fresh baby spinach

- 2 cups of grape tomatoes, halved

- Two cans (15 ounces each) of chickpeas or garbanzo beans, rinsed and drained

- 3/4 cup chopped fresh parsley

- Two green onions, choppedDRESSING:

- 1/4 cup olive oil

- Three tablespoons lemon juice

- 3/4 teaspoon salt

- 1/4 teaspoon garlic powder

- 1/4 teaspoon hot pepper sauce

- 1/4 teaspoon pepper

Instructions

1.   Take an outsized saucepan and convey broth to a boil. Stir in orzo; return to a boil. Reduce heat; simmer, covered, until hard , 8-10 minutes.

2.   Take an outsized pan and add spinach and warm orzo, allowing the spinach to wilt slightly. Add tomatoes, chickpeas, parsley and green onions.

3.   Whisk together dressing ingredients. Toss with salad.

Nutrition

122 calories, 5g fat, 0 cholesterol, 259mg sodium, 16g carbohydrate (1g sugars, 4g fibre), 4g protein. Diabetic Exchanges: 1 starch, one fat.

Roasted Chicken Thighs with Peppers & Potatoes

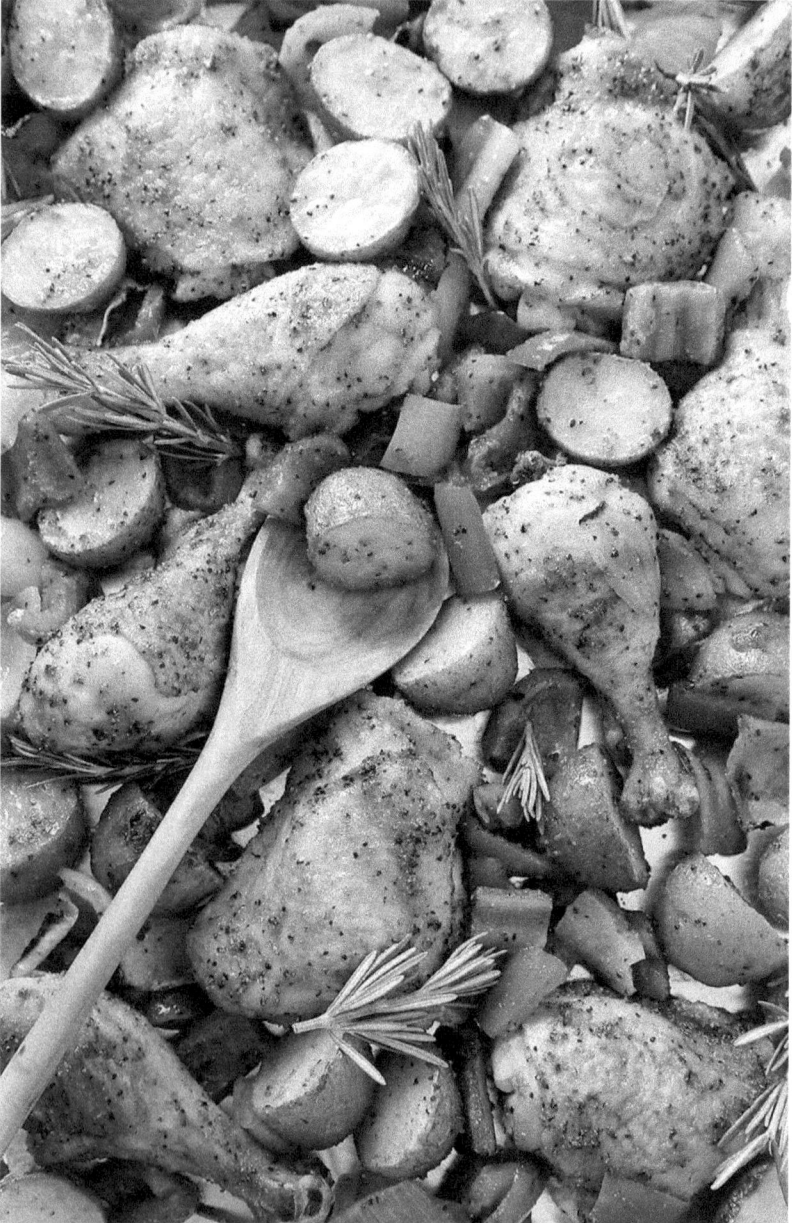

Ingredients

- 2 pounds red potatoes (about six medium)

- Two large sweet red peppers

- Two large green peppers

- Two medium onions

- Two tablespoons olive oil, divided

- Four teaspoons minced fresh thyme or 1-1/2 teaspoons dried thyme, divided

- Three teaspoons minced fresh rosemary or one teaspoon dried rosemary, crushed, divided

- Eight boneless skinless chicken thighs (about 2 pounds)

- 1/2 teaspoon salt

- 1/4 teaspoon pepper

Instructions

1.   Preheat oven to 450°. Cut potatoes, peppers and onions into 1-in. Pieces. Place vegetables during a roasting pan.Drizzle with one tablespoon oil; sprinkle with two teaspoons each thyme and rosemary and toss to coat. Place chicken over greens. Brush chicken with remaining oil; sprinkle with remaining thyme and rosemary. Drizzle vegetables and chicken with salt and pepper.

2.   Roast until a thermometer inserted in chicken reads 170° and green vegetables are tender 35-40 minutes.

Nutrition Facts

308 calories, 12g fat (3g saturated fat), 76mg cholesterol, 221mg sodium, 25g carbohydrate (5g sugars, 4g fibre), 24g protein. Diabetic Exchanges: 3 lean meat, one starch, one vegetable, 1/2 fat.

Spiced Split Pea Soup

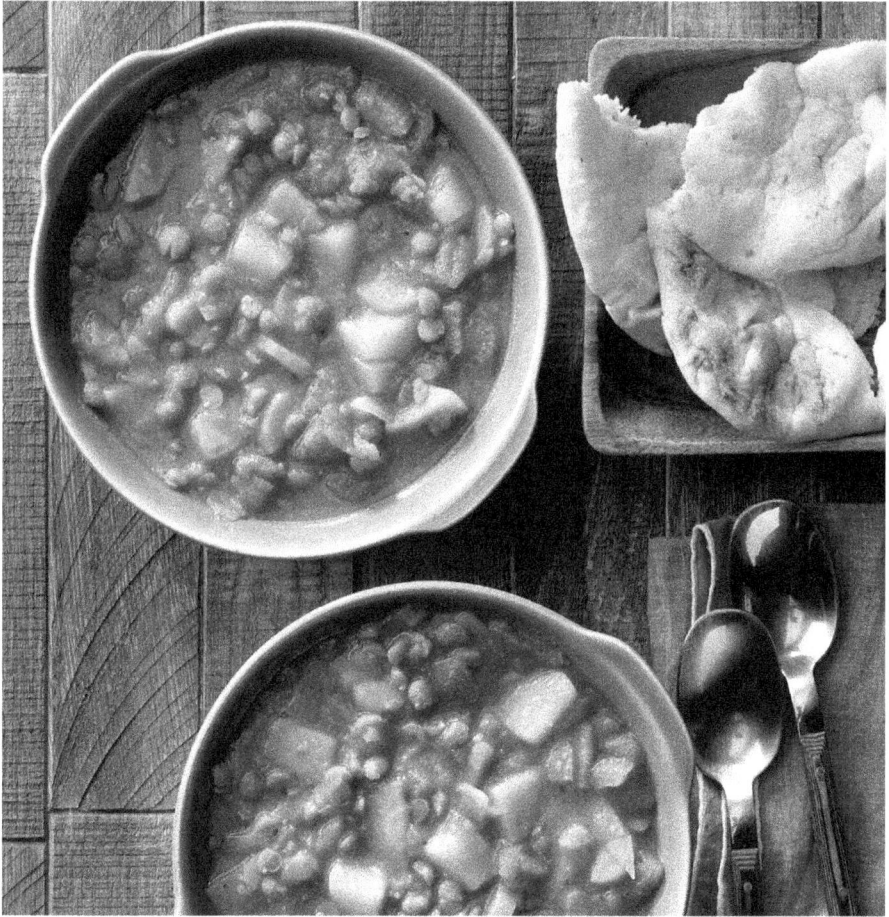

Ingredients

- 1 cup dried green split peas

- Two medium potatoes, chopped

- Two medium carrots, halved and thinly sliced

- One medium onion, chopped

- One celery rib, thinly sliced

- Three garlic cloves, minced

- Three bay leaves

- Four teaspoons curry powder

- One teaspoon ground cumin

- 1/2 teaspoon coarsely ground pepper
- 1/2 teaspoon ground coriander

- One carton (32 ounces) reduced-sodium chicken broth
  One can (28 ounces) diced tomatoes, undrained

Instructions

1. In a 4-qt. Slow cooker combines the primary 12 ingredients. Cook, covered, on low until peas are tender, 8-10 hours.
2. Stir in tomatoes; heat through. Discard bay leaves.

Nutrition Facts

139 calories, 0 fat (0 saturated fat), 0 cholesterol, 347mg sodium, 27g carbohydrate (7g sugars, 8g fibre), 8g protein. Diabetic Exchanges: 1 starch, one lean meat, one vegetable.

Escarole and Bean Soup

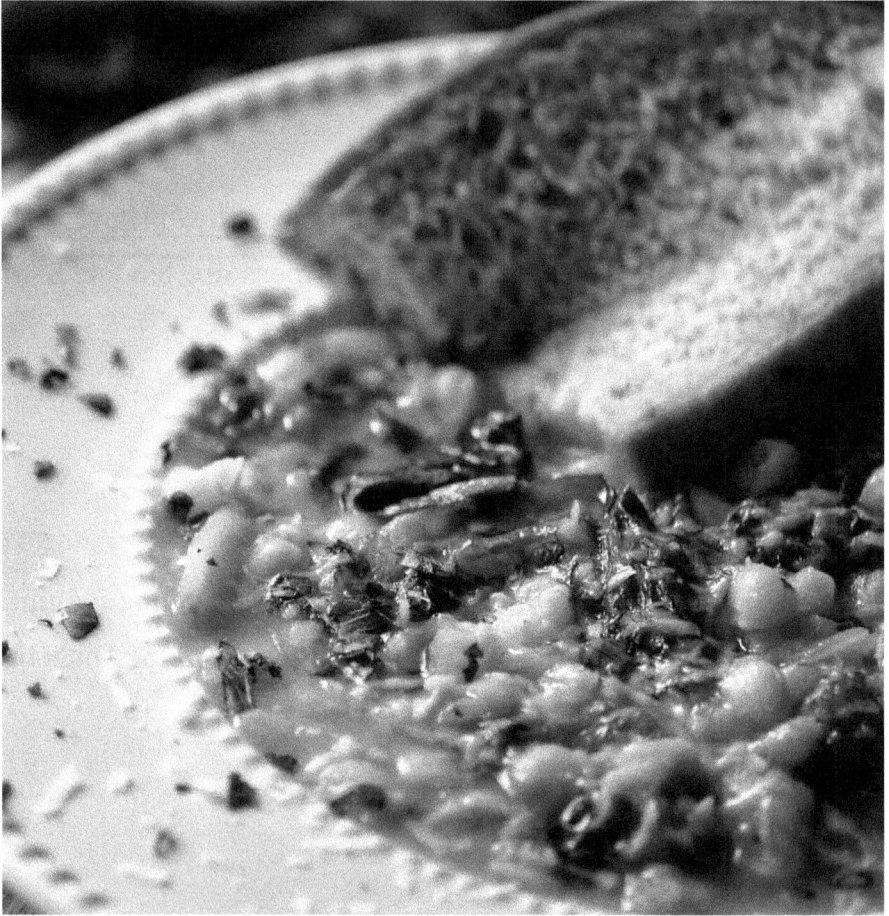

Ingredients

- Two tablespoons olive oil

- Two chopped garlic cloves

- 1 pound of escarole, chopped

- Salt

- 4 cups of low-salt broth chicken

- 1 can of cannellini beans

- 1 (1-ounce) piece of Parmesan

- Freshly ground black pepper
- Six teaspoons extra-virgin olive oil

Directions

1.   Heat vegetable oil during a big heavy pot at normal heat. Add the garlic and sauté till fragrant, for 15 seconds. Add the escarole and sauté till wilted, for 2 min. Add salt. Add the chicken, beans, then Parmesan cheese. Cover and simmer till the beans are heated through, approximately five minutes — season with salt and pepper, to taste.

2.   Ladle the soup into six bowls. Sprinkle one teaspoon extra-virgin vegetable oil over each. Serve with crusty bread.

Italian Pasta Salad with Tomatoes and Artichoke Hearts

SmartPoints value: Green plan - 5SP, Blue plan - 5SP, Purple plan - 5SP

Total Time: 28 min, Prep time: 18 min, Cooking time: 10 min, Serves: 6

Nutritional value: Calories - 296.2, Carbs - 47.3g Fat - 8.2g, Protein - 8.7g

The best time to make this pasta salad is at the height of summer when fresh tomatoes are at their glorious, unrivalled peak. Make sure you use the ripest, juiciest tomatoes you can find. Tomato juices will add a delicious flavour to the dressing.

The chopped artichoke hearts will add a briny taste to every bite. Cellentani pasta is the macaroni formed into a spiral shape, also known as cavatappi. If you can't find that variety, feel free to use whatever type you can get, although short kinds of pasta like penne, rotini, and macaroni would work best. Turn this into a meal by adding some grilled or sautéed chicken or shrimp.

Ingredients

- Tomato(es) (fresh) - 1 pound(s), ripe beefsteak or Campari, chopped (3 cups)

- Bell pepper(s) (uncooked) - 2 item(s), small, yellow and orange, diced (1 ½ cups)

- Artichoke hearts without oil (canned) - 14 oz, drained, roughly chopped

- Basil (torn or coarsely chopped) - 1 cup(s)

- Red wine vinegar - 2 Tbsp

- Olive oil (extra virgin) - 2 Tbsp

- Table salt - ½ tsp, with extra for cooking pasta

- Black pepper - ½ tsp, freshly ground

- Garlic powder - ¼ tsp, or more to taste

- Pasta (uncooked) - 6 oz, cellentani recommended (2 cups)
  Parmesan cheese (shredded) - ⅓ cup(s), or shaved, divided

Instructions

1.   Combine artichoke hearts, basil, tomatoes, peppers, vinegar, oil, salt, pepper, and garlic powder in a large bowl, then toss to coat. Allow the pasta to stand while cooking, occasionally tossing.

2.   Boil a pot of well-salted water and cook the pasta according to package directions. Drain and rinse it with cold water, then drain again.
3.   Add the pasta to the bowl with tomato mixture and toss to coat. Add all but two Tbsp Parmesan and toss again.
4.   Serve the pasta salad with the remaining cheese sprinkled over to the top.

Tofu-veggie Kebabs with Peanut-sriracha Sauce

SmartPoints value: Green plan: 7SP, Blue plan - 3SP, Purple plan - 3SP

Total Time: 41 min, Prep time: 35 min, Cooking time: 6 min, Serves: 4

Nutritional value: Calories - 144.7, Carbs - 9.5g Fat - 8.9g, Protein - 8.8g

Are you planning to go meatless at your next barbecue? Veggie kebabs are your perfect companion. These broccoli, tofu, and radish favorites offer a delicious option for a vegetarian, vegan, or someone who demands a fresher take on the usual cookout. Put the kebabs together quickly in the kitchen.

Then, brush them with an easy-to-make savory sauce before placing them on the grill. Powdered peanut butter makes this nutritious sauce that adds loads of flavor to the favorites.

Cooking them takes about six minutes, and they are perfect for your next picnic. You can pair them with a fresh side salad to increase the vegetable tally.

Ingredients

- Broccoli (uncooked) - 10 oz, florets (about 4 cups)

- Cooking spray - 4 spray(s)

- Firm tofu (rinsed and drained) - 28 oz

- Table salt - ½ tsp

- Radish(es) (fresh, trimmed and halved) - 8 medium

- Lime juice (fresh) - 1½ Tbsp

- Peanut butter (powdered) - 6 Tbsp

- Water - 4½ Tbsp

- Ketchup - 3 Tbsp

- White miso - 3 Tbsp, (low-sodium)

- Soy sauce (low-sodium) - 1½ Tbsp

- Sriracha hot sauce - 1½ tsp

- Sesame oil (toasted) - 1½ tsp

- Sesame seeds (unsalted toasted) - 1 Tbsp

Instructions

1.   Soak up to eight 10-inches bamboo skewers in a shallow dish containing water for at least 20 minutes (or use metal skewers).

2.   Put water in a large saucepan and bring it to a boil over high heat. Add salt and radishes to the pan and cook for 5 minutes.
3.   Add broccoli and cook for 1 minute more. Drain a colander into the saucepan and its content, then Dash the vegetables under cold water until it is cool to the touch. Drain it properly; Pat it dry with paper towels.
4.   Dry out the tofu blocks with paper towels and cut each block into 12 even cubes.
5.   To prepare the sauce, stir the water and powdered peanut butter together in a medium bowl to form a smooth, loose paste.
6.   Add lime juice, ketchup, miso, Sriracha, soy sauce, and oil, then stir to mix.
7.   To prepare kebabs, thread two broccoli florets, two radish halves, and three tofu cubes on each skewer.

8.   Apply medium-high heat to a grill. Brush the kebabs with sauce on one side and lightly coat with cooking spray off the heat.
9.   Place the kebabs on the grill, sauce side down and cook for 2-3 minutes.
10.   Brush the other side with the sauce, flip it and cook for another 2-3 minutes.
11.   Remove the kebabs from the grill and brush them with extra sauce, then sprinkle them with sesame seeds before serving.

Crockpot Beef Stew

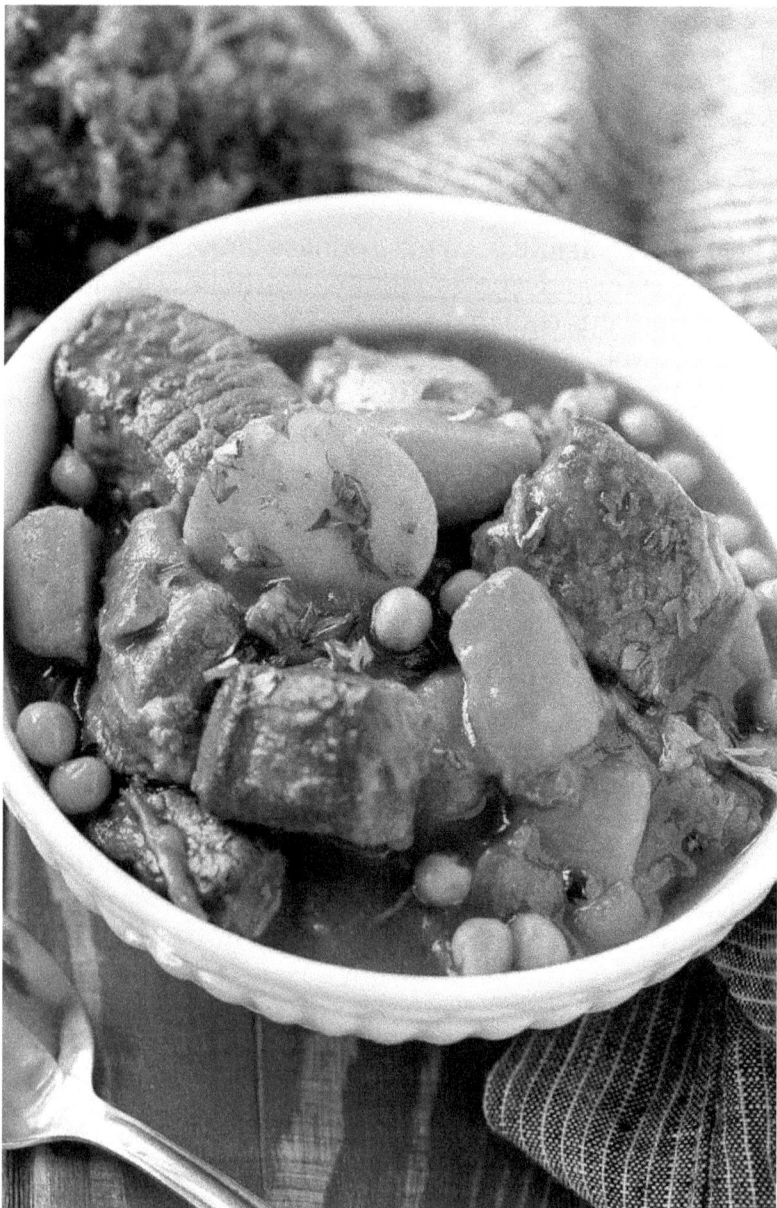

Using a crockpot for stew is not just comfortable but also guarantees that I don't burn it to the bottom of the pot. I love the fact that I can refrigerate my stew in the crockpot overnight, and the next morning, all I need to do is put it in the crockpot base and turn it on.

If you are thinking of a fitting meal for a cold winter evening, give this beef stew a try. It is one of the highly-rated meals over time. I believe the taste will leave you wanting more.

SmartPoints value: Green plan - 6SP, Blue plan - 6SP, Purple plan - 6SP

SmartPoints value: Green plan - 6SP, Blue plan - 6SP, Purple plan - 6SP

Total Time: 1hr 15min, Prep time: 15 min, Cooking time: 1hr, Serves: 8

Nutritional value: Calories – 343, Carbs – 23.5g, Fat – 17.3g, Protein – 22.2g

Ingredients

- Beef chuck roast - 2 lb

- Russet potatoes (2-in diameter) - 4 medium

- Carrots - 4 medium

- Onion - 1 large

- Garlic - 4 cloves

- Onion soup mix - 1 packet

- Fat-free beef broth - 8 cups

- Celery stalks (chopped) - 4 medium

- Add salt and pepper (to taste)

Instructions

1. Chop the roast into pieces (1 inch)

2. Cut peeled potatoes into slices (1/2 inch)
3. Cut peeled carrots into equal chunks (1/2 inch)
4. Cut onion into large pieces
5. Mix the beef, celery, carrots, potatoes, onion, garlic, onion soup mix and beef broth inside the crockpot
6. Add seasoning to taste (salt and pepper)
7. Cook till it's ready
8. This meal is easy to prepare. All you need to do is give it a try and enjoy it.

.